TABLE OF CONTENTS

Top 20 Test Taking Tips

1. Carefully follow all the test registration procedures
2. Know the test directions, duration, topics, question types, how many questions
3. Setup a flexible study schedule at least 3-4 weeks before test day
4. Study during the time of day you are most alert, relaxed, and stress free
5. Maximize your learning style; visual learner use visual study aids, auditory learner use auditory study aids
6. Focus on your weakest knowledge base
7. Find a study partner to review with and help clarify questions
8. Practice, practice, practice
9. Get a good night's sleep; don't try to cram the night before the test
10. Eat a well balanced meal
11. Know the exact physical location of the testing site; drive the route to the site prior to test day
12. Bring a set of ear plugs; the testing center could be noisy
13. Wear comfortable, loose fitting, layered clothing to the testing center; prepare for it to be either cold or hot during the test
14. Bring at least 2 current forms of ID to the testing center
15. Arrive to the test early; be prepared to wait and be patient
16. Eliminate the obviously wrong answer choices, then guess the first remaining choice
17. Pace yourself; don't rush, but keep working and move on if you get stuck
18. Maintain a positive attitude even if the test is going poorly
19. Keep your first answer unless you are positive it is wrong
20. Check your work, don't make a careless mistake

Triage

Emergency Intake

Rapid visual assessment: Sick vs. not sick

Sick vs. not sick is a rapid visual assessment method used for initial triage and is usually completed within less than a minute based on clinical indications. The primary purpose is to classify as "sick" those who appear unstable and require immediate attention and as "not sick" those who appear stable and have no or less severe illness/injury and whose care can be delayed. Decisions are made based on knowledge about expected injuries from different types of accidents, the mechanism of injury (auto accident, gunshot wound, fall), and nature of sickness that might suggest possible diagnoses. Clinical indicators to evaluate include:

- Vital signs: Pulse and respiration.
- Mental status: Alert, confused, responsive, non-responsive, disoriented.
- Circulation: Skin signs include cyanosis, pallor, erythema, and edema.
- Body position: Sitting, standing, prone, supine, distorted.
- Evidence of trauma, mechanism of injury (trauma): Bleeding, open wounds, fractures.
- Nature of medical complaints (illness): Pain, dizziness, and dyspnea.

Patients initially classified as "not sick" may be reclassified at any time their conditions change.

Pediatric Assessment Triangle (PAT)

The Pediatric Assessment Triangle (PAT) is a method used to provide a first general impression of a child's state of health and/or illness. Each parameter is evaluated as normal or abnormal with abnormal findings requiring further assessment per the primary and secondary surveys.

Pediatric Assessment Triangle (PAT)	
Appearance	Note the child's tone, ability to interact, response to environmental stimuli, consolability, gaze, general appearance, and speech or crying. Other descriptors include: listless, responding poorly, lethargic, poor muscle tone (rigid, floppy), staring.
Breathing	Note the degree of difficulty associated with breathing, including any abnormal or adventitious breath sounds, sternal retraction, nasal flaring, bobbing of head, and positioning (such as the need to sit upright to breathe). Other descriptors include: stridor, grunting, crackles, wheezing, and absent breath sounds.
Circulation	Note the color of skin and any abnormalities, such as mottling, pallor, bleeding, or cyanosis. Other descriptors include: Circumoral cyanosis, peripheral cyanosis.

Life-threatening illnesses/injuries

Epidural hemorrhage - Hemorrhage is always a concern with head trauma because even injuries that appear slight can result in vascular rupture, leading to hemorrhage between the skull and the brain. There are two types of hemorrhage that often occur from head trauma: epidural and subdural. Epidural hemorrhage is bleeding between the dura and the skull, pushing the brain downward and inward. The hemorrhage is usually caused by arterial tears, so bleeding is often rapid, leading to severe neurological deficits and respiratory arrest. Initially, the body compensates by rapidly absorbing cerebrospinal fluid and decreasing blood flow, but the compensatory measure is soon overwhelmed. The most common site is the parietotemporal region, forcing the medial part of the temporal lobe under the tentorial edge, compressing nerves and vessels. This type of injury usually results from unintentional falls and rarely from child abuse. It is not common in children <4 years. Diagnosis in small children is often delayed because of nonspecific symptoms.

Subdural hemorrhage - is bleeding between the dura and the cerebrum, usually from tears in the cortical veins of the subdural space. It tends to develop more slowly than epidural hemorrhage and can result in a subdural hematoma. If the bleeding is acute and develops within minutes or hours of injury, the prognosis is poor. Subacute hematomas that develop more slowly cause varying degrees of injury. Subdural hemorrhage is a common injury related to birth trauma but otherwise is usually caused by child abuse, although it can result from coagulopathies or aneurysms. Symptoms of acute injury may occur within 24–48 hours, but subacute bleeding may not be evident for up to 2 weeks after injury. Chronic hemorrhage occurs primarily in the elderly. Symptoms vary and may include bradycardia, tachycardia, hypertension, and alterations in consciousness. Subdural taps may suffice for infants, but some infants and older children will require surgical evacuation of the hematoma.

Subarachnoid hemorrhage - is a common injury after trauma and may result from childbirth (one of the most common causes) or from abuse (shaken impact syndrome) along with subdural hematoma. While less common in children than adults, subarachnoid hemorrhage can also occur from rupture of a berry aneurysm or an arteriovenous malformation (AVM). However, there are a number of disorders that may be implicated: neoplasms, sickle cell disease, infection, hemophilia, and leukemia. The first presenting symptom in infants may be seizures, and usually symptoms are similar to those of subdural hematoma. Older children may complain of severe headache, nausea and vomiting, nuchal rigidity, palsy related to cranial nerve compression, retinal hemorrhages, and papilledema. Symptoms will worsen as intracranial pressure rises. Treatment includes:

- Identifying and treating underlying cause.
- Anti-seizure medications (such as Dilantin®) to control seizures.
- Antihypertensives.
- Surgical repair if indicated.

Hypovolemic shock - is the most common affecting children, occurs when intravascular volume decreases by 15–25% because of traumatic blood loss; plasma loss through increased capillary permeability causing fluid to shift from the vascular system to the interstitium; or dehydration, which may result from diarrhea or vomiting. Characteristics include decreased preload, increased afterload, and no change in contractibility. The decrease in intravascular volume results in less venous return to the heart and decreased ventricular filling, resulting in decreased preload (stretch) and increased afterload (vascular resistance) which reduces stroke volume, cardiac output, and tissue perfusion, causing hypotension. Treatment includes:

- Ventilatory support: Intubation with positive pressure ventilation and oxygen.
- Fluid replacement: Crystalloid solution in boluses of 10–20 mL/kg over 10–15 minutes, repeated as necessary. Colloids containing proteins (albumin) may be given or blood products if shock is related to blood loss and hematocrit is markedly decreased.
- Vasopressor (dopamine) to improve cardiac output.
- Vasodilators (nitroprusside, amrinone, or hydralazine) when blood volume adequate.

Limb-threatening injuries - Any injury to an extremity should be assessed for limb-threatening conditions:

- **Pulse**: The limb should be assessed for pulse to evaluate the integrity of the vasculature. If no pulse is palpable, then Doppler assessment is indicated.
- **Color/temperature:** Pallor or cyanotic changes indicate impaired circulation. With impaired circulation, the limb may feel cooler than an unaffected limb.
- **Sensation**: Numbness, tingling, or lack of sensation often indicate nerve damage and severe injury that may be limb threatening.

Some types of injuries increase risk to the limb, including partial amputations, gunshot wounds, displaced fractures, and knee dislocations, which can result in severe neurovascular impairment with damage to the popliteal artery and occlusion in up to half of incidences. The injury may cause a clot to form so that even after reduction, impairment may occur. Compression injuries increase risk of compartment syndrome, which can rapidly impair circulation. With any limb-threatening condition, immediate identification and intervention is essential to preserve the limb.

Assigning triage acuity levels

Emergency Severity Index (ESI) - is a 5-level method of triage that evaluates the patient's condition and need for resources. The 5 levels are based on decision point questions and include:

- **1:** Unstable and needs resuscitation/lifesaving interventions immediately. Diagnoses include: cardiac arrest, respiratory arrest or severe distress, SPO2 <90, severe trauma, overdose, hypovolemia, anaphylaxis, hypoglycemia with mental status change, signs of MI, marked bradycardia.
- **2:** High-risk patient needs time-sensitive treatment (usually within 10 minutes) to prevent threat to life or organ. Diagnoses include chest pain, indications of stroke, fever in immunocompromised, suicidal/homicidal ideation, staff member needle stick.
- **3:** Patient requires ≥2 resources. Patient is stable and may wait an hour or so for treatment. Note: Resources include laboratory tests, imaging, IV fluids, parenteral medications, nebulizer treatment, referral to specialist, and simple procedures (suturing, catheter insertion), or complex procedures (conscious sedation). Complex procedures are considered equivalent to 2 resources.
- **4:** Patient requires 1 resource.
- **5:** Patient requires no resources.

Emergency Severity Index (decision points) - includes 4 questions or decision points used to assign patients to Levels 1 through 5.

- **Is the patient dying?** If yes, the patient is classified as ESI 1, ABCs assessed, and lifesaving procedures instituted: BVM, intubation, surgical airway, C-PAP, Bi-PAP, cardioversion, pacing, defibrillation, chest needle compression, pericardiocentesis, IV/blood transfusion, reversal agents. If the patient is not dying, then the next question is posed.
- **Should the patient not wait?** Assessments include determining if the patient is at high risk, confused/disoriented, and/or in severe pain or distress. If yes, the patient is classified as ESI 2. If not, the next question is posed.
- **How many resources are needed?** This evaluation depends on knowledge of usual treatment for presenting symptoms. Patients are classified at level 3, 4, or 5 based on expected needs.

- **What are the vital signs?** This includes pulse, respiration, oxygen saturation, and temperature (for children <3). If VS are unstable, patients classified as level 3 are elevated to level 2.

S.T.A.R.T. - Simple Triage and Rapid Treatment is a method of triage used when there are multiple casualties that must be assessed rapidly and classified for treatment. Colored tags are applied to identify status. Classification is based on sequential evaluation of respirations, perfusion, and mental status (RPM):

- **Green: Minor.** Patient may have injuries, but RPMs are intact, and patient can wait for assistance.
- **Blue: Deceased.** Head is repositioned, but if respirations do not occur, CPR is not started, but the triage person moves on to the next patient.
- **Red: Immediate.** If breathing resumes after head repositioning, respirations are >30 (estimated, not counted), there is no radial pulse, capillary refill >2 seconds, or if patient is unconscious or cannot follow simple commands, classify as "Immediate."
- **Delayed: Other conditions.** Classify as "Delayed" if patient is able to follow simple commands and needs are not immediate.

Three-level and four-level triage

Three-level triage is still used in some emergency departments with some variations. The criteria for assignment may vary somewhat as well. Generally, the 3 levels include:

- **Critical/Immediate/Emergent:** These patients have life-threatening conditions that require immediate resuscitation or intervention to prevent death or severe morbidity and have priority for treatment.
- **Urgent:** These patients have serious injuries that require treatment, but care can be delayed for a few minutes while those with more serious injuries are treated.
- **Less urgent/Non-urgent:** These patients are assigned the lowest priority because their injuries are not life threatening.

Four-level triage is similar. The primary difference is the addition of a "Resuscitation" category separate from those who otherwise require critical care. For example, a patient with cardiac arrest would be classified as "Resuscitation" and a myocardial infarct as "Emergent." Various color-coding systems, sometimes specific to a facility, may be used.

Identifying decontamination need

Most exposures to hazardous materials, such as chemicals and biologicals, and the need for **decontamination** are identified prior to transfer to a hospital. Children are most likely to become exposed as a result of large spills of hazardous material or from contact with pesticides or other materials stored or used in the home. If the hazardous material is identified, a reference guide, such as those supplied by NIOSH should be accessed to determine correct procedures, as these may vary depending on the material. If a child appears with unidentified powder or particles on the body or wet clothing from spills, exposure to hazardous material should be suspected. Most hazardous materials are non-reactive to water, so the first step is generally to remove clothing and shower thoroughly, preferably outside the facility. If no outside shower is available or the child is too ill or young to shower independently, then the staff must follow protocol in decontaminating the child.

Resource needs based on volume

In emergency medicine, **resources** include laboratory tests, imaging, IV fluids, parenteral medications, nebulizer treatment, referral to specialist, simple procedures (suturing, catheter insertion), or complex procedures (conscious sedation). Treatments that are NOT considered resources include immunizations, oral medications, prescriptions, dressings, crutches, point-of-care testing, history, and physical examination. Information gleaned from ESI triage system can help to determine needs according to volume and triage level. Average ED visits per level include:

- Level 3 (needing 2 or more resources): 30–40%.
- Level 4 (needing 1 resource): 20%.
- Level 5 (needing 0 resources): 35%.

Using these percentages and the volume of patients, one can estimate the need for resources. However, not all facilities, such as level 1 trauma center, fit this pattern of distribution, so each facility should undertake research to determine the actual utilization of resources per trauma category.

Pharmacological agents used for asthma:

- **β-Adrenergic agonists** - -Include both long-acting and short-acting preparations used for relaxation of smooth muscles and bronchodilation, reducing edema and aiding clearance of mucus. Medications include salmeterol (Serevent), sustained release albuterol (Volmax ER®) and short-acting albuterol (Proventil®) and levalbuterol (Xopenex®). Side effects include insomnia, tremors, increased wheezing, and anxiety.
- **Anticholinergics** - Aid in preventing bronchial constriction and potentiate the bronchodilating action of β-Adrenergic agonists. The most-commonly used medication is ipratropium bromide (Atrovent®). Side effects include cough, headache, nausea, and allergic reactions.
- **Corticosteroids** - Provide anti-inflammatory action by inhibiting immune responses, decreasing edema, mucus, and hyper-responsiveness. Because of numerous side effects, glucocorticosteroid are usually administered orally or parentally for 5 days (prednisone, prednisolone, methylprednisolone) and then switched to inhaled steroids. If a child receives glucocorticoids for more than 5 days, then dosages are tapered. Inhaled corticosteroids include beclomethasone (Vanceril®), budesonide (Pulmicort®) and fluticasone propionate (Flovent®). Side effects include immunosuppression, Cushing's syndrome, weight gain, bruising, acne, facial swelling.
- **Methylxanthines** - -Are generally contraindicated unless a child is critically ill, in which case they appear to have a role in improving pulmonary function and decreasing need for mechanical ventilation. Medications include aminophylline and theophylline. Side effects include insomnia, anxiety, tremor, tachycardia, nausea, vomiting, and diarrhea.
- **Magnesium sulfate** - Is used to relax smooth muscles and decrease inflammation. If administered intravenously, it must be given slowly to prevent hypotension and bradycardia. Inhaled, it potentiates the action of albuterol. Side effects include allergic reaction, diarrhea, and stomach pain.
- **Heliox** - (Helium-oxygen)-Is administered to decrease airway resistance with airway obstruction, thereby decreasing respiratory effort. Heliox improves oxygenation of children on mechanical ventilation.
- **Leukotriene inhibitors** - Are used to inhibit inflammation and bronchospasm for long-term management. Medications include montelukast (Singulair®). Side effects include headache, flu-like symptoms, abdominal pain, and cough.

HSS

Hypertonic saline solution (HSS) has a sodium concentration higher than 0.9% (NS) and is used to reduce intracranial pressure/cerebral edema and treat traumatic brain injury. Concentrations usually range from 2% to 23.4%. The hypertonic solution draws fluid from the tissue through osmosis. As edema decreases, circulation improves. HSS also expands plasma, increasing CPP, and counteracts hyponatremia that occurs in the brain after injury and causes increased ICP.

Administration:

- **Peripheral lines: HSS <3% only.**
- **Central lines**: HSS ≥3%.

HSS can be administered continuously at rates varying, depending on age of child, usually 5 mL/kg/dose. Rate must be carefully controlled. Fluid status must be monitored to prevent hypovolemia, which increases risk of renal failure. Boluses (typically 30 mL of 23.4%) may be administered over 15 minutes for acute increased ICP or transtentorial herniation.

Laboratory monitoring includes:

- **Serum sodium** (every 6 hours): Maintain at 145–155 mEq/L. Higher levels can cause heart/respiratory/renal failure.
- **Serum osmolality** (every 12 hours): Maintain at 320 mOsml/L. Higher levels can cause renal failure.

Mannitol

Mannitol is an osmotic diuretic that increases excretion of both sodium and water and reduces intracranial pressure and brain mass, especially after traumatic brain injury. Mannitol may also be used to shrink the cells of the blood-brain barrier in order to help other medications breach this barrier. Mannitol is administered per intravenous infusion:

- 0.25–2 g/kg (age-dependent) in a 15% to 25% solution over one-half to one hour.

Cerebral spinal fluid pressure should show decrease within 15 minutes. Fluid and electrolyte balances must be carefully monitored as well as I & O and body weight. Concentrations of 20% to 25% require a filter. Crystals may form if the mannitol solution is too cold and the mannitol container may require heating (in 80° C water) and shaking to dissolve crystals, but solution should be cooled to ≤body temperature prior to administration. Mannitol cannot be administered in polyvinylchloride bags as precipitates form. Side effects include fluid and electrolyte imbalance, nausea, vomiting, hypotension, tachycardia, fever, and urticaria.

Antidysrhythmics

Paroxysmal Supraventricular tachycardia	Adenosine. **Digoxin (Lanoxin®)** affects the conduction system and may cause bradycardia, heart block, nausea and vomiting, and CNS depression. **Verapamil (Calan®, Verelan®)** affects the conduction system and may cause decreased BP, bradycardia, and heart failure.
Sinus tachycardia	Esmolol (Brevibloc®)
Premature ventricular contractions	**Lidocaine** affects the ventricles and may cause CNS toxicity with nausea and vomiting. Procainamide
Ventricular tachycardia	Lidocaine. Amiodarone (Cordarone®, Pacerone®). Procainamide
Ventricular fibrillation	Lidocaine
Atrial fibrillation	Digoxin (Lanoxin®) Diltiazem (Cardizem®, Tiazac®) **Ibutilide (Corvert®)** affects the conduction system and rarely has side effects. **Amiodarone (Cordarone®)** affects the atria and ventricles and may cause decreased BP, and adverse hepatic effects.
Atrial flutter	Digoxin (Lanoxin®) Diltiazem (Cardizem®, Tiazac®) Ibutilide (Corvert®) Verapamil (Calan®, Verelan®) Amiodarone (Cordarone®) Procainamide

Pulmonary pharmacology Antimicrobials

Antibiotics	Used for treatment of respiratory infections, including pneumonia. Medications are used according to the pathogenic agent and may include macrolides (usually for use with children over 5), such as azithromycin (Zithromax®), erythromycin (E-Mycin®). Antibiotics used for children <5 include 3rd generation cephalosporins, such as ceftriaxone (Rocephin®) and cefotaxime (Claforan®). Ampicillin and 2nd generation cephalosporins (Zinacef®, Ceftin®) are also used. Side effects include rash, nausea, vomiting, and diarrhea.
Antimyco-bacterials	Used for treatment of TB and other mycobacterial diseases. Medications include isoniazid (Laniazid®, Nydrazid®), ethambutol (Myambutol®), rifampin (Rifadin®), streptomycin sulfate, and pyrazinamide. Side effects include rash, flushing, nausea, vomiting, joint pain, and optic neuritis.
Antivirals	Used to inhibit replication of virus early in a viral infection. Effectiveness decreases as time passes because replication process has already begun. Medications include ribavirin (Virazole®) and

	zanamivir (Relenza®). Side effects include dizziness, muscle pain, fatigue, flu-like symptoms, headache, dry mouth, nausea, vomiting or diarrhea.

Triage Interventions

Protective splinting

Protective splinting for accidental injuries	
Shoulder	The arm should be placed in a sling with the wrist/hand above the level of the elbow.
Humerus	A rigid splint should be applied on the lateral humerus and the arm secured in a sling across the chest with swath binder.
Elbow	The elbow is splinted in position found. If straight, splint from axilla to wrist along medial aspect with splint tied in place. If bent, place rigid splints from upper arm to wrist and support in sling.
Forearm	Place rigid splint, or SAM splint, on both sides of arm with thumb upward from palm and extending past elbow. Then, support in sling with swath binder about body.
Pelvis & hip	Provide firm backboard and avoid lifting legs.
Femur	Rigid splints on both sides of leg can be used or buddy splinting if necessary. Traction splints are preferred but usually only available with EMS.

RICE(R) therapy

Rest-The person should immediately stop doing the activity that caused the problem in order to avoid further damaging the area.
Ice-Ice or cold compresses should be applied for 15–20 minutes/hour for the first 24–48 hours to reduce swelling.
Compression-An Ace bandage or similar dressing should be used to apply gentle pressure and prevent and/or reduce swelling.
Elevation-The injured area should be elevated above the level of the heart, often by using pillows to elevate the body part.

Referral should be made to appropriate specialist for care as needed.

Eye wash procedures

- **Flush-**Use an emergency eyewash (fixed or portable) with 2 spray heads that deliver irrigant (water or NS at 60–95°F) at the rate of 0.4 gal/minute (gpm). Bend over the flush station with eyelids held open by the thumbs and index fingers with spray aimed at the base of the nose (inner canthus to outer canthus) rather than the eyeball. Flush eyes for at least 15 minutes for caustic chemicals. Remove contact lenses as soon as possible (before or shortly after initial flushing).
- **Irrigation-**Position patient with head elevated to about 20°. Place protective drape and emesis basin beside patient's head on side to be flushed. Turn patient to side so solution will flow into basin. Fill bulb syringe with irrigant, usually NS. Hold eyelid open with thumb and index finger. Irrigate with tip about one-half inch above eye, with flow aimed at the lower

conjunctival sac from inner canthus to outer. Flush for about 1 minute unless otherwise indicated.

Analgesia: Equianalgesic

Equianalgesic is a comparison of doses of different analgesics that provide equivalent analgesia/sedation. Children must be monitored carefully with all analgesics. Intravenous analgesics usually take effect within 15–30 minutes while oral medications take twice as long. Dosage must be calculated according to age and weight:

Drug	Parenteral	Oral
Morphine sulfate	10 mg.-Infant starts at 0.05 mg/kg and child at 0.1 mg/kg.	30 mg.-Child dosage varies according to preparation.
Dilaudid	1.5mg.-Infant and child starts at 0.015 mg/kg.	7.5 mg.-Child dosage varies according to preparation.
Fentanyl	100 mcg.-Infant and child starts at 0.5–2 mcg/kg.	Varies (patches)
Demerol	75 to 100 mg.-Infant and child starts at 1–1.5 mg/kg.	300 mg. -Not recommended for child. Used for shivering not for analgesia.
Codeine	120 mg.-Not recommended for child.	200 mg.-Child dosage varies according to preparation.
Vicodin	--	30 mg.-Child dosage varies according to preparation.

Acetaminophen

Drug	Dosage	Side effects
Acetamin-ophen	Dosages may be repeated every 4 hours to max of 5 in 24 hours. Dosage based on 10–15 mg/kg with adult dosing at 12 years: **0–3 mths**: 40 mg (to max of 200 mg/24 hr). **2–3 yrs**: 120 mg (to max of 600 mg/24 hr). **6–8 yrs**: 320 mg (to max of 1600 mg/24 hr). **11 yrs**: 480 mg (to max of 2400 mg/24 hr)	Allergic response with itching, rash, edema. Liver toxicity with overdose

NSAIDS

Drug	Dosage	Side effects
Choline magnesium trisalicylate	<37 kg/81.5 lb: 50 mg/kg/d divided in 2 doses >37 kg/81.5 lb: 2250 mg/d divided in 2 doses	Tinnitus. GI irritation with nausea, vomiting, diarrhea, constipation, epigastric discomfort
Ibuprofen	<6 months to 12 years: 5–10 mg/kg every 6–8 hours (to maximum of 40 mg/kg/day) 12–18 years: 200–400 mg every 4–6	Nausea, vomiting, diarrhea. Gastrointestinal irritation with ulcerations and bleeding. Bleeding nephritis. Retention of fluid

	hours to maximum of 2400 mg/day	
Naprosyn	>2 years: 20 mg/kg/day divided in 2 doses	Same as ibuprofen
Tolmetin	>2 years: 20 mg/kg/day divided in 3–4 doses	Same as ibuprofen

Pain management

Non-pharmacologic Methods of Managing Pain	
Behavioral contracting	Use rewards (stickers, privileges) for compliance and cooperation. Write up contract that outlines expectations and rewards for compliance and cooperation (such as not hitting during dressing changes).
Distraction	Encourage games, radio, TV, play, music, deep breathing, blowing bubbles, and reading books.
Guided imagery	Encourage child to think of a pleasant event and describe it, concentrating on all aspects of the event (sounds, feelings, tastes, colors, smells).
Positive thinking	Teach child to make positive statements: "I will feel better soon." Teach child to counter focus on negative experiences with positive thoughts: "The shot only lasts a few seconds."
Relaxation exercises	Infant, small child: Hold and rock or sway back and forth. Older child: Use progressive relaxation by tightening and relaxing parts of body.

Length-based resuscitation tape

Length-based resuscitation tape is used to estimate weight according to length in infants and small children. The measurement is taken from head to heel with the child in supine position. The results are used to determine dosages of drugs and sizes of equipment. Dosages of common emergency drugs are printed on the tape for different lengths although some calculations for volume and concentration may be required. The marked tape is usually extended alongside the child. A straight edge should be used when possible to increase accuracy at both ends. The Broselow® tape is commonly used by emergency departments and first responders. Lengths are divided by colors into different "zones," related to length/estimated weight. In some emergency departments, pediatric carts are color coded to correspond to the zones on the tape. It's important to use the tape properly, with the top at the head of the child, colored red (for head) on the Broselow® tape.

5 rights of drug administration

Five rights of drug administration	
Right drug	Evaluate drug orders in terms of diagnosis and pediatric contraindications. Ensure orders are generated by those with prescriptive rights. Contact prescriber if drug seems inappropriate or incorrect.
Right dose	Use single-dose medications if possible. If calculating a dose to prepare from a dose other than that ordered, check calculations with a second person. Pour liquid drugs into medicine cups at eye level. Draw medication slowly into syringes and check for bubbles.Double check dosage order before administration and consider age of child and appropriateness.
Right client	Use two identifiers, including the identifying name band and one other.

Right route	Check route as per order. Notify prescriber if ordered route is that recommended. Check label of medication for route.
Right time	Administer according to established schedule—within 30 minutes of scheduled time and following directions, such as "before meals."

Safety related to medication errors

There are about 7000 deaths yearly in the United States attributed to **medication errors.** Studies indicate that there are errors in 1 in 5 doses of medication given to patients in hospitals. A caring environment is one in which patient safety is ensured with proper handling and administering of medications:

- Avoiding error-prone abbreviations or symbols. The Joint Commission has established a list of abbreviations to avoid, but mistakes are frequent with other abbreviations as well. In many cases, abbreviations and symbols should be avoided altogether or restricted to a limited approved list.
- Preventing errors from illegible handwriting. Handwritten orders should be block printed to reduce change of error.
- Instituting bar coding and scanners that allow the patient's wristband and medications to be scanned for verification.
- Providing lists of similarly named medications to educate staff.
- Establishing an institutional policy for administering of medications that includes protocols for verification of drug, dosage, and patient as well as educating the patient about the medications.

Antidysrhythmics

Antidysrhythmics include a number of drugs that act on the conduction system, the ventricles and/or the atria to control dysrhythmias. There are 4 classes of drugs that are used as well as some that are unclassified:

- **Class I**: 3 subtypes of sodium channel blockers (quinidine, lidocaine, procainamide)
- **Class II**: β-receptor blockers (esmolol, propranolol)
- **Class III**: Slows repolarization (amiodarone, ibutilide)
- **Class IV**: Calcium channel blockers (diltiazem, verapamil)
- **Unclassified** (Adenosine)

Antidysrhythmics	
Supraventricular tachycardia	**Adenosine** affects conduction system and may cause transient flushing, decreased BP, and shortness of breath. **Diltiazem (Cardizem®, Tiazac®)** affects conduction system and may cause bradycardia, AV block, and decreased BP. **Esmolol (Brevibloc®)** affects the conduction system and may cause decreased BP, bradycardia, and heart failure. **Propranolol (Inderal®)** affects conduction system and may cause bradycardia, heart block, and heart failure. **Procainamide** affects the atria and ventricles and may cause decreased BP and ECG abnormalities (widening of QRS and QT).

Assessment

History and Physical

Primary survey

Primary survey - ABCDE survey

- **A-Airway-**Check airway for obstruction. Open airway with head tilt chin maneuver (lift chin with one hand and apply pressure to forehead with the other) or if trauma is present, the jaw thrust (stabilize cervical spine and pull mandible forward).
- **B-Breathing-**Look, listen, and feel for breathing for up to 10 seconds. If not breathing, institute bag-valve-mask (BVM) ventilation followed by nasotracheal or orotracheal intubation if no response.
- **C-Circulation-**Provide basic life support (BLS). Check pulse: Carotid pulse in children >1 year, brachial pulse in infants, umbilical pulse in neonates. Begin CPR: 120 compressions per minute in neonates and 100 per minute for infants and children. Defibrillation. If no response, institute Advanced Cardiovascular Life Support (ACLS).
- **D-Disability-**Evaluate neurological status: Pupillary response, level of alertness, Glasgow Coma Scale, CT for suspected stroke, blood glucose level and naloxone for suspected narcotic overdose.
- **E-Exposure/ Environmental control-**Remove clothes, check body for lesions, rashes, trauma, and maintain thermoregulation.

Secondary survey

Secondary survey	
History	Question medical problems, current medications, onset of illness or injury, allergies, time of last meal, and pregnancy status when applicable.
Head	Examine eyes, ears, nose, throat, skull, and skin for lacerations and bruises.
Neck	Note carotid pulses, stiffness, bruit, jugular venous distention and trauma.
Chest	Complete inspection, palpation, percussion, and auscultation. Note hyperresonance, dullness, adventitious sounds, or absent breath sounds.
Heart	Note rhythm, heart sounds, and murmurs.
Abdomen	Complete careful examination with supporting laboratory (blood counts) and imaging assessment (ultrasound, radiograph, CT, MRI) as needed.
Rectal, genital, perineal	Perform examination if indicated.
Musculo-skeletal	Inspect and palpate all extremities for fractures, lacerations, dislocations, motor function, sensation, and pulses with supporting imaging as indicated. Multiple trauma patients should have pelvis x-ray.
Neurological	Assess level of consciousness and complete evaluation of pupils

	and cranial nerves, reflexes, motor function, and sensory level with supporting imaging, such as CT scans. Note evidence of spinal cord injury.

American Spinal Injury Association Impairment Scale (ASIA)

The American Spinal Injury Association Impairment Scale (ASIA) is used for initial assessment of a child with SCI and on an ongoing basis during treatment to assess changes. S4-S5 controls anal sensation and sphincter contraction, so anal examination is important in determining level of impairment:

A	Complete impairment with no motor or sensory function, including at S4-S5. No anal sensation or sphincter contraction.
B	Incomplete impairment with sensory function but no motor function. Anal sensation is present but not sphincter contraction.
C	Incomplete impairment with motor function maintained below neurological level and >50% of key muscles below neurological level have <3 muscle grade.
D	Incomplete impairment with motor function maintained below neurological level and >50% of key muscles below neurological level have ≥3 muscle grade.
E	Normal motor and sensory functions.

Assessment of heart sounds: S1, S2

Auscultation of **heart sounds** can help to diagnose different cardiac disorders. Areas to auscultate include the aortic area, pulmonary area, Erb's point, tricuspid area, and the apical area. The normal heart sounds represent closing of the valves.

The first heart sound (S1) "lub" is closure of the mitral and tricuspid valves (heard at apex/left ventricular area of the heart).

The second heart sound (S2) "dub" is closure of the aortic and pulmonic valves (heard at the base of the heart). There may be a slight splitting of the S2.

The time between S1 and S2 is systole and the time between S2 and the next S1 is diastole. Systole and diastole should be silent although ventricular disease can cause gallops, snaps, or clicks and stenosis of the valves or failure of the valves to close can cause murmurs. Pericarditis may cause a friction rub.

Additional heart

Additional heart sounds	
Gallop rhythms	S3 occurs after S2 in children and young adults but may indicate heart failure or left ventricular failure in older adults (heard with patient lying on left side). S4 occurs before S1 and occurs with ventricular hypertrophy, such as from coronary artery disease, hypertension, or aortic valve stenosis.
Opening snap	Unusual high-pitched sound occurring after S2 with stenosis of mitral valve from rheumatic heart disease.
Ejection click	Brief high-pitched sound occurring immediately after S1 with stenosis of the aortic valve.

Friction rub	Harsh, grating sound heard in systole and diastole with pericarditis.
Murmur	Sound caused by turbulent blood flow from stenotic or malfunctioning valves, congenital defects, or increased blood flow. Murmurs are characterized by location, timing in the cardiac cycle, intensity (rated from Grade I to Grade VI), pitch (low- to high-pitched), quality (rumbling, whistling, blowing) and radiation (to the carotids, axilla, neck, shoulder, or back).

Glasgow coma scale

The **Glasgow coma scale (GCS)** measures the depth and duration of coma or impaired level of consciousness and is used for postoperative assessment. The GCS measures three parameters: Best eye response, best verbal response, and best motor response, with a total possible score that ranges from 3 to 15. The same scale is used with slight modifications for infants.

Eye opening	**4**: Spontaneous. **3**: To verbal stimuli. **2**: To pain (not of face). **1**: No response
Verbal	**5**: Oriented (Infant: Smiles, exhibits appropriate interactions). **4**: Conversation confused, but can answer questions (Infant: crying but consolable) **3**: Uses inappropriate words (Infant: Moaning, sometimes inconsolable). **2**: Speech incomprehensible (Infant: Inconsolable, agitated). **1**: No response
Motor	**6**: Moves on command (Infant: Moves spontaneously or with purpose). **5**: Moves purposefully to respond to pain. **4**: Withdraws in response to pain **3**: Decorticate posturing (flexion) in response to pain. **2**: Decerebrate posturing (extension) in response to pain. **1**: No response

Injuries/conditions are classified according to the total score:

- **3–8** Coma; ≤ 8 Severe head injury
- **9–12** Moderate head injury
- **13–15** Mild head injury

Normal cardiac rates

Normal cardiac rates can vary widely from one child to another, so it's important to understand the normal range in order to determine if the child has an abnormal pulse. Rates will also vary depending upon whether the child is awake, asleep, or active. Pulse rate should be taken with a stethoscope; especially for infants and small children, the pulse may be difficult to palpate or count accurately manually. Additionally, this allows assessment for heart murmurs.

Newborn infant	At rest: 100–180 Asleep: 80–160 Active/sick: ≤ 220
1–12 weeks	At rest: 100–220 Asleep: 80–200 Active/sick: ≤ 220
3–24 months	At rest: 80–150 Asleep: 70–120 Active/sick: ≤ 200
2–10 years	At rest: 70–110 Asleep: 60–90 Active/sick: ≤ 200

10–adulthood	At rest: 55–90 Asleep: 50–90 Active/sick: ≤ 200

Normal respiratory rate and temperature

Children's vital signs vary considerably according to age, height, and weight.

- **Respiratory rate:** Newborns breathe about 35 (30 to 60) times per minute and then respirations begin to slow to 30 by age 1 month, dropping to 24 to 30 during ages 1 to 3, and 22 to 34 by age 6. Respiratory rates for children 6 to 12 range from 18 to 30 and then decrease to a rate similar to adults of 12 to 16 between ages 12 and 28.
- **Temperature:** The normal temperature for a child up to 3 years ranges from 37.5°C (99.4°F) at birth to 37.2° (99°F) at 3. The typical "normal" temperature of 37°C (98.6°F) is reached at 5 years, but temperature usually continues to decline to a normal of 36.6°C (97.8°C) by age 13.

Cranial nerve assessment

Cranial nerve assessment	
I. Olfactory (Smell)	Ask the child to smell and identify a substance, such as coffee or soap, with one nostril held closed, and then the other.
II. Optic (Vision)	Test visual acuity and the ability to recognize color. Test each eye separately. Red desaturation is tested by having the child look at a red object with first one eye and then the next to determine if the color looks the same with both eyes or is dull with one eye.
III. Oculomotor (Eye muscles and pupil response)	Using a penlight, check eyes for size, shape, reaction to light and accommodation. Check eyes for rotation and conjugate movements while the child follows a light or toy with the eyes. Examine the lids for ptosis.
IV. Trochlear (Eye muscles: upward movement)	Check eye movement by having the child follow a moving finger with the eyes on the vertical plane.
V. Trigeminal (Chewing muscles and sensory)	Ask the child to close the eyes for the sensory examination and instruct the child to indicate when part of the face is stroked (light stroke with cotton). Stroke the forehead, cheek, and jaw. Then, examine the same areas for sharp or dull. Observe the eyes for blinking and tearing, but touching the cornea with cotton or other items should be avoided as it can cause abrasion. Assess the jaw muscles by having the child hold the mouth open as well as by palpating the muscles on each side to determine if they are equal in size and strength.
VI. Abducens (Eye muscles: lateral movement)	Ask the child to follow the finger from the 1 o'clock position clockwise to the 11 o'clock position. At the horizontal and vertical axis, check the eyes for deviation or nystagmus, which may occur normally only in the extreme lateral position.
VII. Facial nerve (Facial expression, tears, taste, and saliva)	Usually, only the motor portion is evaluated for nerve VII, and taste is examined with testing of cranial nerve IX, but one can test the ability to discriminate between salt and sugar. Assess motor functions by asking the child to frown, smile, puff out the

	cheeks, and wrinkle the forehead. Observe the muscles for symmetry. Ask the child to hold the eyes tightly closed while the examiner attempts to open the lids with the thumb on the lower lid and the index finger on the upper lid, using care not to apply pressure to the eye.
VIII. Vestibulocochlear (Balance and hearing)	Check balance with tandem gait and Romberg's test (stand child with eyes closed to determine if the child can maintain balance.) Check hearing by asking the child to close the eyes and then rubbing fingers together or holding ticking watch next to one of the child's ears and then the other. Weber's test may be done to evaluate lateralization and Rinne's test for bone and air conduction. **Weber's test:** Touch a vibrating tuning fork to the top of the head or the forehead and ask the child if sound is equal in both ears. Hearing deficit in one ear suggests sensorineural hearing loss. **Rinne's test:** Hold a vibrating tuning fork on the mastoid bone and measure the time until sound ceases. Then hold the vibrating tuning fork at the external ear. Sound is normally heard twice as long through air as through bone. If there is conductive hearing loss, the sound is heard longer through the bone. If there is sensorineural hearing loss, the sound is heard longer through the air.
IX. Glossopharyngeal (Taste and mouth sensation)	This test is not usually performed unless the child complains of lack of taste or abnormalities of taste. The mouth must be moist for accurate assessment, so the child should drink water if possible before the test and the testing substance should be in solution. The child is tested for recognition of sweet, sour, bitter, and salt.
X. Vagus (Swallowing and gag reflex)	Ask the child to open the mouth and say "aw." The uvula and palate should elevate equally on both sides. The gag reflex is usually tested if the person reports difficulty swallowing or changes in speech. Test the gag reflex by lightly touching the tongue blade to the soft palate. Some children are hyper-responsive, so accurate testing of the gag reflex may be difficult.
XI. Spinal accessory (Muscle movement: sternocleidomastoid and trapezius)	Test these muscular movements by placing the hands along the side of the face and asking the child to turn the face first one side and then the other against resistance to determine if strength is normal and equal. Then, place hands on the child's shoulders and ask the child to shrug the shoulders, elevating them upward, against resistance to determine if the strength is normal and equal.
XII. Hypoglossal (Tongue)	Ask the child to stick out the tongue to determine if it deviates to one side, indicating a lesion on that side of the brain. To determine if there is equal strength on both sides of the tongue, hold a tongue blade against the side of the tongue and ask the child to push against it with the tongue. Check both sides to determine if strength is normal and equal.

Peripheral nerve assessment

A musculoskeletal evaluation should include **peripheral nerve assessment** to determine if injury has impaired nerve function. Nerve function should be assessed for both sensation and movement. Assessment of sensation is done with a sharp or pointed instrument, using care not to prick the skin. The child should feel a slight prick if the sensory function is intact:

- **Median:** The median nerve branches from the brachial plexus, which arises from C5, C6, C7, C8, and T1. The median nerve travels down the arm and forearm, through the carpal tunnel. Sensation is evaluated by pricking the top or distal surface of the index finger. Movement is evaluated by having the child touch the ends of the thumb and little finger together and having the child flex the wrist.
- **Peroneal:** The peroneal nerve branches from the sciatic nerve, which arises from the L4, L5, and S1, S2, and S3 dorsal nerves and travels down the leg. The peroneal nerve enervates the lower leg, foot, and toes. Evaluate sensation by pricking the webbed area between the great and second toe. Evaluate movement by having the child dorsiflex and extend the foot.
- **Radial:** The radial nerve branches from the brachial plexus and enervates the dorsal surface of the arm and hand, including the thumb and fingers 2, 3, and 4. Evaluate sensation by pricking skin in the webbed area between the thumb and the index finger. Evaluate movement by having the child extend the thumb, the wrist, and fingers at the metacarpal joint.
- **Tibial:** The tibial nerve branches from the sciatic nerve. The tibial nerve travels down the back of the leg, through the popliteal fossa at the back of the knee and terminates at the planter surface of the foot. Sensation is evaluated by pricking the medial and lateral aspects of the plantar surface of the foot. Movement is evaluated by having the child plantar-flex the toes and then the ankle.
- **Ulnar:** The ulnar nerve branches from the sciatic nerve and travels down the arm from the shoulder, traveling along the anterior forearm beside the ulna, to the palm of the hand. Sensation is evaluated by pricking the distal fat pad at the end of the small finger. Movement is evaluated by having the child extend and spread all fingers

Examination of the pupils

Examination of the eyes: Pupils
Note size, shape, symmetry, reaction, and accommodation: • Benign anisocoria: slight inequality in size with no other abnormalities • Horner's syndrome (impaired sympathetic nerve impulse): pupil small, regular, reactive to light and accommodation, associated with ptosis • Ocular nerve paralysis: nonreactive dilated pupil, sometimes associated with lateral deviation and ptosis • Tonic pupil: large, regular with reduced or absent reaction to light and slow accommodation • Argyll Robertson (usually associated with syphilis): bilateral small, irregular pupils nonreactive to light but normal accommodation • Dilated, fixed: brain damage, hypoxia, anticholinergic agents and glutethimide poisoning • Small, fixed: pontine hemorrhage, glaucoma eye drops, and narcotic drugs • Surgical abnormalities: iridectomy

Medical and surgical history

The emergency nurse is expected to demonstrate competency in assessment, including **medical and surgical history**, as part of identifying and managing health concerns in infants and children. Complete and accurate documentation of findings is an essential element of the plan of care. **History:** This may be done in the classic manner that begins with a complaint and includes health history, surgical history, review of systems, nutrition, developmental status, family history, and socioeconomic factors that may affect the health issue. This should include detailed information about medical conditions, treatments, and surgery. A problem-oriented history builds upon the classic history by focusing on developmental health problems, functional problems, and diseases, moving from subjective information (history) to objective (physical/laboratory data):

- Developmental assessment includes motor, speech, cognitive, social, and adaptive behaviors.
- Functional assessment includes issues related to basic health behavior patterns, such as diet, sleeping, coping, sexuality, and elimination.
- Diseases are those diagnoses according to the *International Classification of Diseases,* Clinical Modification (ICD-9-CM, used to classify morbidity data), and interventions are planned based on diagnosis.

While the essential elements of assessment and **medical and surgical history** for adolescents are similar to those for infants and children, there are some differences because often the adolescent is providing, or in some cases withholding, information. Additionally, the risk factors associated with adolescence vary from those of infancy or earlier childhood. Assessment should include lifestyle information, such as whether the teenager has been homeless, engaged in high-risk sexual behavior, violence, tobacco use, or drug use. Documenting nutrition, weight concerns, peer relationships, and coping mechanisms can help to identify health concerns. A complete history should include information about medical conditions, treatment, and surgery. Successful assessment includes:

- Listen and show respect for the adolescent.
- Question adolescent/parent cause for concern.
- Interview both the adolescent and the parent(s) alone.
- Observe nonverbal behavior and interactions among children and parents.

Domestic/dating violence

According to guidelines of the Family Violence Prevention Fund, assessment for **domestic/dating violence** should be done for all adolescent patients, regardless of background or signs of abuse. While females are the most common victims, there are increasing reports of male victims of domestic violence, both in heterosexual and homosexual relationships. The person doing the assessment should be informed about domestic violence and be aware of risk factors and danger signs. The interview should be conducted in private (or with parent if children <3 years old). The office, bathrooms, and examining rooms should have information about domestic violence posted prominently. Brochures and information should be available to give to patients. Patients may present with a variety of physical complaints, such as headache, pain, palpitations, numbness, or pelvic pain. They are often depressed and may appear suicidal and may be isolated from friends and family. Victims of domestic violence often exhibit fear of perpetrator (such as a parent, boyfriend, or girlfriend) and may report injury inconsistent with symptoms.

Describe injuries consistent with domestic/dating violence/abuse

Injuries consistent with domestic/dating violence/abuse	
Characteristic injuries	Ruptured eardrum. Rectal/genital injury—burns, bites, trauma. Scrapes and bruises about the neck, face, head, trunk, arms. Cuts, bruises, and fractures of the face
Patterns of injuries	Bathing suit pattern—injuries on parts of body that are usually covered with clothing as the perpetrator abuses but hides evidence of abuse. Head and neck injuries (50%)
Abusive injuries (rarely attributable to accidents)	Bites, bruises, rope and cigarette burns, welts in the outline of weapons (belt marks). Bilateral injuries of arms/legs
Defensive injuries	Back of the body injury from being attacked while crouched on the floor face down. Soles of the feet from kicking at perpetrator. Ulnar aspect of hand or palm from blocking blows

Physical growth and development during infancy

The newborn sleeps about 16 hours/day during the **first month** but is growing and developing.

- **Growth:** Infant loses 5–7% of birth weight and then gains 4–7 ounces/week (about 2 lbs/month). Head circumference increases 1.5 cm/month and length 1.5 cm.
- **Mobility:** The infant makes fists and flexes arms and legs. Reflexes such as Moro, sucking, grasping, startle, rooting, and asymmetric tonic neck are present.
- **Feeding:** About every 2–3 hours with breastfeeding.
- **Urine/feces:** Urination is about 8 times/day. Breastfed babies may have frequent loose stools or may skip 2–3 days. If bottle-fed, stools are usually more firm. Color varies (yellow, tan, green, brown).
- **Sensory:** Follows items in line of vision and often prefers faces and contrasting geometric designs. Vision is somewhat blurry with ability to focus at about 8–15 inches. Color distinction is poor. Babies hear well and respond with startle reflex. Sense of smell is strong.
- **Communication:** Infant signals distress with crying, gagging, and arching body and responds to comfort measures.

During **months 2–4,** the infant continues to sleep much of the time but is often awake for periods in the morning, afternoon, and evening.

- **Growth:** Gains 5–7 ounces/week and 1.5 cm length/month and 1.5 cm head circumference/month. Posterior fontanel closes.
- **Mobility:** Loses grasp reflex and hands start to stay open and grasp. Able to lift head while prone or supine and turn from side to side. Can roll stomach to back by 4 months. Moro reflex fades. Plays with hands. Can be pulled to standing position.
- **Feeding:** Needs about 2 oz/lb/24 hours, usually feeding every 4 hours.
- **Urine/feces:** Urine is about 5–6 times/day. Stools vary from one each feeding to every 2–3 days, but usually are more firm and regular.
- **Sensory:** Can focus at about 12 inches and follows objects 180° with eyes.

- **Communication:** Crying differentiates to show hunger, pain, frustration. Infant can smile indiscriminately by 2 months and socially responsive smile by 3 months. Child shows preference for mother and may turn from strangers.

During **4–6 months** the child sleeps about 10–11 hours at night, with 2–3 daytime naps (total 15 hours).

- **Growth:** Doubles weight by 5–6 months, gains 5–7 oz/week.
- **Mobility:** Infant can roll over and roll from back to side by 6 months; can hold head up at 90° and turn head in both directions when sitting or lying. Can sit with support for 10–15 minutes. Grasp improves and may hold bottle and play with feet. By 6 months, can pick up items and move items from one hand to the other. Manipulates and mouths objects and watches objects fall.
- **Feeding:** Still having about 2 feedings at night and every 4 hours during the day, 1.5 oz/lb/24 hours.
- **Urine/feces:** Urination and defecation becoming regular.
- **Sensory:** Eyes focus well; follows items/people with eyes.
- **Communication:** Vocalizes more and mimics tones. Squeals and laughs. Yells with anger. Vocalizes to get attention and recognizes family members.

During **6–8 months** the child begins to have more waking hours, sleeping 10–11 hours with 2 naps.

- **Growth:** Growth slows. Gains 3–5 oz/wk and 1 cm in length/month.
- **Mobility:** Can sit alone by 8 months. Can stand supported and bounces on legs. Starting to use pincer grasp. Easily manipulates and moves objects. Most birth reflexes have faded. Bangs objects together and mouths objects freely.
- **Feeding:** Starting to take solid foods (cereal, vegetables, and fruit) 2–3 times daily as well as breastfeeding/bottle-feeding 3–5 times daily. Teething biscuits, graham crackers, and Melba toast may be introduced.
- **Urine/feces:** Stool larger with solid foods. Urinating 5–6 times daily.
- **Sensory:** Watches and listens actively, turning head to sounds and to follow objects.
- **Communication:** Increased babbling and mimicking of sounds, including two syllable sounds and vowels, such as "mama" or "dada" but doesn't use intentionally. Has babbling conversations. May be fearful of strangers.

During **8–10 months,** the child continues to sleep about 10–11 hours at night and usually sleeps through the night, with 2 naps in the daytime.

- **Growth:** Gains 3–5 oz/wk and 1 cm in length/month.
- **Mobility:** Uses pincer grasp well and can pick up small objects. Crawls or creeps readily. Can sit up and by 10 months can pull to standing position by holding onto furniture.
- **Feeding:** Meat introduced. Breastfeeding or bottle-feeding 3–4 times daily with 3 meals. Egg yolks only may be introduced. Will enjoy finger foods, such as meat sticks.
- **Urine/feces:** Fairly regular.
- **Sensory:** Watches and listens freely, attentive.
- **Communication:** Babbles and may be able to say one or two words besides "mama" or "dada." Understands basic vocabulary, such as "no" and "cookie." Babbling follows speech-like rhythm when "talking."

During **10–12 months**, the child continues to sleep 10–11 hours at night with 2 naps in the daytime.

- **Growth:** Gains 3–5 oz/week and 1 cm/month. Head and chest circumference are equal. Birth weight tripled by 12 months.
- **Mobility:** Can make marks on paper with pens or crayons. Fits objects through holes. Can stand alone and walk holding onto furniture. Can sit from standing position.
- **Feeding:** Breastfeeding or bottle-feeding 3–4 times daily and starting with "sippy" cup. Eating solid foods, both prepared baby foods and soft home-cooked foods. Enjoys finger foods and may resist being fed.
- **Urine/feces:** May smear feces. Holding urine for longer periods of time, especially girls.
- **Sensory:** Watches and listens, engaging in activities.
- **Communication:** Understands many words. Uses "mama" and "dada" intentionally and may use a few other words. Plays patty-cake and peek-a-boo games. Enjoys repetition.

Between **1 and 2,** the child is growing in size and independence.

- **Growth:** Gains 8 oz/month and 3–5 in/year. Anterior fontanel closes.
- **Mobility:** Begins with first steps and by 2 walks and runs and can go up and down stairs. Scribbles on paper, throws toys, and learns to stack blocks. Begins independent exploration of environment.
- **Diet:** Child eats 3 meals and 2–3 snacks daily. Whole cow's milk can be taken after 1 year, 2–3 cups daily. Some may breastfeed. Child can consume wide range of foods.
- **Toileting:** Between 18–24 months, some children show an interest in potty training.
- **Communication:** Begins with one word and grows. Learns names for common objects and begins trying to communicate with simple words leading to short sentences around 2 with vocabulary of 30–50 words. May show apprehension with strangers and anger with temper tantrums.

The **2–3 year old** makes significant changes over the course of a year.

- **Growth:** Gains 3–5 lb/year and 3.5–5 in/year.
- **Mobility:** Can run steadily, jump on two feet, and climb. Scribbling becomes more intentional and can draw simple shapes. Makes effort to color in the lines. Able to undress at 2 and dress at 3. Can throw a ball overhand. Plays side by side and begins to interact with others.
- **Diet:** Can switch to lowfat milk, 2–3 cups daily along with a regular well-balanced meal of meat, fruits, vegetables, and grains. Should limit fruit juice to 2–4 oz/day because of high sugar content. Should not be receiving bottle feedings.
- **Toileting:** Most children become potty-trained sometime during this year.
- **Communication/cognition:** Begins to talk in short 3-word sentences and to understand rules. Begins to use pronouns (I, me, you) and can talk about feelings. Usually knows at least 5 body parts and colors and can categorize by size (big, little).

Physical growth and development during preschool years

Between **3–6**, the child moves from being a toddler to a child.

- **Growth:** Gains 3–5 lb/yr and 1.5–2.5 in/year. Most growth occurs in long bones as child increases in stature and proportionate head size decreases.
- **Mobility:** Becomes increasingly adept, drawing various shapes, coloring in the lines, using scissors to cut along lines. Can brush teeth. Can tie shoes by 6. Able to climb, run, jump, balance, and ride tricycle or bicycle with training wheels. Interacts with others.

- **Diet:** Eats 3 meals with snack and can manage spoon, fork, and knife independently by age 6.
- **Communication/cognition:** Becomes increasingly verbal and social and commands a large complex vocabulary by 6. Understands concepts of right and wrong, good and bad, and can lie. Learns letters and numbers and by age 6 is beginning to read. May focus on one thing to the exclusion of others.

Physical growth and development during school age years

During the school years **(ages 6 to 12),** children go through many changes.

- **Dental:** Children lose deciduous teeth and begin acquiring permanent teeth.
- **Height and weight:** These should progress slowly and steadily, gaining an average of 2 inches each year, beginning at about 45 inches at 6 and attaining about 59 inches at 12. Weight usually doubles during this time from 46 pounds at 6 to 88 pounds at 12. Boys and girls are similar in size but by 12, some girls will be undergoing pubertal changes and may gain height and weight over boys.
- **Proportions:** The body becomes slimmer and better proportioned with an increase in muscle mass and decrease in fat. In relation to height, head circumference decreases, leg length increases, and waist circumference decreases. Facial characteristics change.
- **Body systems:** Systems mature with respirations and heart rate decreasing. Bladder capacity is usually better in girls than boys. Muscles strengthen and bones begin to ossify. Physical variation increases with age.

Physical growth and development problems during school-age years

During the years of **6–12,** routine health assessments should be done at ages 6, 8, 10, 11, and 12 to determine if there are developmental delays or problems, which may include:

- **6 years:** Peer problems, depression, cruelty to animals, poor academic progress, speech problems, lack of fine motor skills, and inability to catch a ball or state age.
- **8 years:** No close friends, depression, cruelty to animals, interest in fires, very poor academic progress with inability to do math, read, or write adequately and poor coordination.
- **10 years:** No team sports and poor choices in peers (gangs), failure to follow rules, cruelty to animals and interest in fires, depression, failure to understand causal relationships, poor academic progress in reading, writing, math, and penmanship, and problems throwing or catching.
- **12 years:** Continuation of problems at 10 years with increasing risk-taking behaviors (drinking, drugs, sex) and continued poor academic progress in reading, following directions, doing homework, and organization.

Physical growth and development issues for early adolescence

Early adolescence, **11–14,** is a transitional time for children as their hormones and their bodies go through changes. Children mature at varying rates, so there are wide differences. Emotions may be labile, and the child may feel isolated and confused at times, trying to find an identity. Peers take on more influence and the child may challenge the values of the family. Children may have much anxiety about their bodies and sexuality as secondary sexual characteristics develop. Developmental concerns include:

- Delayed maturation

- Short stature (female)
- Spinal curvature (females)
- Poor dental status (caries, malocclusion)
- Chronic illnesses, such as diabetes
- Lack of adequate physical activity
- Poor nutrition, anorexia, obesity
- Concerns about sexual identity
- Negative self-image, depression
- Lack of close friends, fighting or violent episodes, lack of impulse control
- Poor academic progress with truancy and failure to complete assignments

Normal growth and development issues for middle adolescence

In middle adolescence, ages **15–17**, most body changes have occurred, and there is less concern about this but more concern about the image they are projecting to others. Girls may worry about weight and boys about muscle development. Teenagers are interested in sexuality and many begin sexual experimentation. There is strong identification with peer groups, including codes of dress and behavior, often putting individual at odds with family. Developmental concerns include:

- Spinal curvature (females) and short stature (males)
- Lack of testicular maturation/ persistent gynecomastia
- Acne
- Anorexia, obesity
- Sexual experimentation, multiple partners, and unprotected sex
- Sexual identification concerns
- Depression, poor self-image
- Lack of adequate exercise, poor nutrition, and poor dental health
- Chronic diseases
- Experimentation with drugs and alcohol and problems with authority figures
- vvLack of peer group identification, gang association
- Poor academic progress, failing classes, truancy, attention deficits and disruptive class behavior, poor judgment and impulse control

Normal growth and development issues for late adolescence

Late adolescence, **18–21,** is the time when adolescents begin to take on more adult roles and responsibilities, entering the world of work or going to college. Most have come to terms with their sexuality and have a more mature understanding of people's motivations. Some young people will continue to engage in high-risk behaviors. Many of the problems associated with middle adolescence may continue if unresolved, interfering with the transition to adulthood. Developmental concerns include:

- Failure to take on adult roles, no life goals or future plans
- Low self-esteem, lack of impulse control
- Lack of intimate relationships, sexual identification concerns
- Gang association
- Continued identification with peer group or dependence on parents
- High-risk sexual behavior, multiple partners and unprotected sex
- Poor academic progress or ability
- Psychosomatic complaints, depression

- Poor nutrition, obesity, anorexia
- Poor dental health
- Chronic disease
- Lack of exercise

Maturity assessment

A **maturity assessment** should be part of the examination for children and adolescents to determine their level of sexual, dental, and skeletal maturity. Skeletal maturity is usually assessed by measurements of the hand and wrist as well as weight/height for age. Skeletal maturity and chronological age may differ. For example, if the chronological age is 14.3 and the skeletal age is 15.5, this would be expressed as 15.5–14.3 = SA +1.2. Another method is to divide the skeletal age by the chronological age: a score >1.0 equates with advanced skeletal maturity and <1.0 a delay in skeletal maturity.

The most common assessment tool for sexual maturity is Tanner's 5 stages of assessment. This tool assesses maturity for both males and females, based on direct observation of breasts and genitals.

Females: breast development, onset of menses, and pubic hair distribution
Males: Penis and testes development and pubic hair distribution

Normal hearing developmental characteristics

Hearing deficits may be identified very early by careful observation of developmental characteristics in infants and children. **Normal hearing** responses include:

- **≤3 months:** Positive Moro (startle) reflex to sound. Noise disturbs sleep, and reacts to sounds by opening eyes or blinking.
- **3–6 months:** Comforts at sound of parent's voice and tries to emulate sounds. Looks in the direction of sound.
- **6–12 months:** Begins to vocalize more with cooing and gurgling with different inflections. Responds to name and simple words and looks in the direction of sound.
- **12–18 months:** Begins first words about 12–15 months and imitates sounds, follows vocal directions, and points to familiar items when asked.
- **18–24 months:** More verbal with about half of vocabulary understandable and knows about 20–50 words. Points to body parts or familiar objects when asked.

Language milestones

While children develop at different rates, there are a number of **language milestones** of developmentally appropriate communication for infants and toddlers.

- **5–6 weeks:** Vocalizations usually small and throaty, sometimes during crying
- 2 months: Single vowel sounds (ah, oh, oo, eh)
- **3 months:** Gurgling, laughing, and some consonant sounds (n, k, g, b, p)
- 8 months: Add consonants (t, d, w) and may combine syllables ("mama") although may not attach meaning
- **10 months:** Understand simple words, such as "no" and "mama"
- **12 months:** Say a few words with comprehension, such as "mama," "dada," and can imitate some animal sounds

- **13–15 months:** Have a 4- to 6-word expressive vocabulary but understand many more words and can point to indicate a desire for something, such as a toy
- **16–18 months:** Use 7- to 20-word vocabulary and point to 5 body parts
- **20 months:** Combine 2 words
- **24 months:** Understand 300 words and uses 2- to 3-word sentences

Customizing assessment for children with special needs

- Children may present in the ED with a variety of special needs, so initial assessment should include determining what special needs a child may have and then addressing them.
- **Mentally challenged children** (Down syndrome): Ask caregiver about the child's level of understanding and comfort measures that might distract or ease the child's anxiety. Talk to the child in a soothing manner.
- **Autistic children:** Ask caregiver about those things that trigger anxiety/meltdown in the child and ask caregiver to help support the child. Ask before touching, and touch only as necessary. Explain procedures, especially if child is high functioning.
- **Vision-impaired children:** Maintain a dialogue explaining activities and procedures, such as "I'm going to feel your tummy." Allow the child to touch equipment, such as a stethoscope, when possible.
- **Hearing-impaired children:** Ask about degree of hearing loss and methods the child uses to communicate. Use a sign language interpreter if appropriate or ensure hearing aids are in place and functioning. Use pictures of treatments or procedures if possible.

Using developmentally appropriate communication

Children, even toddlers, should always receive an explanation of treatment or other aspects of care, but the explanations should be given with **developmentally appropriate communication**, avoiding technical terms the child may not understand. Short explanations are better for small children as they may become very anxious. If more detailed explanations are needed for the parents, these explanations should be given away from the child.

Avoid	**Use**
Shot, injection, bee sting, needle stick	Medication under the skin
Incision, cut	Special opening
Pain	Hurt, "owie," or other term used by the child
Take temperature	See how warm you are
Monitor	TV/Computer screen
Stool, feces	Use child's term (poop, caw-caw)
Urine	Pee-pee
Gurney	Rolling bed
X-ray	Special pictures
Catheter	Tube
Anesthetize, deaden	Make sleepy, numb
Treat	Fix, make better

Identifying caregivers' perception of child's baseline

During times of emergency, a child's caregivers may be stressed, but the nurse must have information regarding the caregivers' perception of the **child's baseline status**, especially with infants and younger children or those who are developmentally delayed. The nurse should ask specific questions rather than very general questions, such as "What behavior or activity is normal for your child?" Questions relate to the child's age, but those for infants and young children should include:

- Height and weight
- Diet: If nursing or bottle-fed, include frequency and duration of nursing or ounces of milk per feeding. Question number of meals daily and typical diet and eating habits.
- Mobility: Varies by age, but include ability to grasp, roll, turn, sit up, walk, run, and manipulate items.
- Elimination: Include bowel and urinary output, problems, habits, routine, and continence. If infant, include number of diapers daily.
- Sensory: Include age-appropriate indications of hearing and vision.
- Communication: Include age-appropriate communication, such as vocalizing, babbling, saying words, saying sentences, comprehension.

Child abuse and reporting requirements

About 5 million cases of suspected **child abuse** are reported in the United States each year. In accordance with the Child Abuse Prevention and Treatment and Adoption Act Amendments (1996) and the Model Child Protection Act, all states have instituted mandatory reporting of child abuse. The clinical nurse specialist should be knowledgeable about the statutes in the state of practice, but medical personnel are mandatory reporters and must report the following:

- Child abuse or neglect that places the child at risk of harm (physical or emotional), death, or exploitation.
- Sexual abuse including rape, molestation, prostitution, incest, or engaging in any type of sexually explicit behavior.
- While some statutes mandate reporting mere suspicion, others mandate only reporting specific knowledge. Regardless, there is criminal and civil liability involved if child abuse is not reported, and most states provide immunity for reporters. Thus, the best course is to report even suspicions to child protective services or the police, according to the state requirements.

Behavioral and physical signs of physical abuse in children

Children rarely admit to being abused and, in fact, typically deny it and attempt to protect the abusing person. Therefore, the critical care nurse must often rely on physical and behavioral signs to determine if there is cause to suspect **abuse**.

- **Behavioral indicators:** The child may be overly compliant or fearful with obvious changes in demeanor when a parent/caregiver is present. Some children act out with aggression toward other children or animals. Children may become depressed or suicidal or present with sleeping or eating disorders. Behaviors may become increasingly self-destructive as the child ages.
- **Physical indicators:** The type, location, and extent of injuries can raise suspicion of abuse. Head and facial injuries and bruising are common, as are bite or burn marks. There may be hand prints or grab marks, unusual bruising, such as across the buttocks. Any bruising, swelling, or tearing of the genital area and the identification of sexually transmitted diseases are also causes for concern.

Signs of neglect and lack of supervised care in children.

While some children may not be physically or sexually abused, they may suffer from profound **neglect or lack of supervision** that places them at risk. Indicators include:

- Appearing dirty and unkempt, sometimes with infestations of lice, and wearing ill-fitting, torn clothing and shoes
- Being tired and sleepy during the daytime
- Having excessive medical or dental problems, such as extensive dental caries
- Missing appointments and not receiving proper immunizations
- Being underweight for their current stage of development

Neglect can be difficult to assess, especially if the critical care nurse is serving a homeless or very disadvantaged population. Home visits may be needed to ascertain if there is adequate food, clothing, or supervision, and this may be beyond the scope of care provided by the critical care nurse. Thus, suspicions should be reported so that social workers can arrange a follow-up assessment of the home environment.

Pain

Pain assessment (NIPS)

Pain assessment of neonates and infants depends on careful observation of a number of different characteristics. The **Neonate/Infant Pain Scale (NIPS)** assesses 6 areas with a score >3 indicating pain. Five areas are scored 0–1, depending upon the degree of stress. Crying, which is often the most indicative of pain, is scored 0–2.

	0	**1**	**2**
Expression	Rested, normal	Negative, tight muscles, grimace	
Crying	None	Intermittent moaning, whimper	Loud crying
Respiratory patterns	Relaxed, normal	Irregular breathing, tachypnea, holding breath, gagging	
Upper extremities	Relaxed, random move-ment	Tense, rigid or rapid extending and flexing	
Lower extremities	Relaxed, random move-ment	Tense, rigid or rapid extending and flexing	
Arousal state	Awake or asleep, random leg move-ments	Restless, fussing, thrashing about	

Pain assessment of children 1–7 (CHEOPS)

The **Children's Hospital Eastern Ontario Pain Scale (CHEOPS)** is used for children 1–7 and is based on scores of 6 different characteristics with scores of 0–2 except for crying, which is scored 0–3. A score >4 indicates pain.

	0	1	2	3
Crying		Not crying	Silent crying, moaning	Loud Cry
Express-ion	Happy	Neutral	Grimacing	
Verbal	Does not com-plain	Quiet	Complain about pain or pain and other things	
Torso		Inactive relaxed	Tense, moving, shivering, and sitting upright	
Upper extrem-ities		Not touching reaching for injury	Gently touching, grabbing injury or arms restrained	
Lower extrem-ities		Relaxed, random move-ment	Restless, tense, kicking, kneeling, or legs restrained	

Note: Children over 7 may be able to describe pain or indicate pain according to facial expression scale, but this may be difficult for younger children.

Assessment of pain for cognitively impaired (NCCPC). Vocal, Social Facial

The **Non-communicating Children's Pain Checklist** (NCCPC) is designed for children 3 to 8 who are cognitively impaired but may be used for children recovering from anesthesia (modified version). The checklist contains 7 categories with sublistings that are each scored: 0 (not occurring), 1 occurring occasionally, 2 occurring fairly often, 3 occurring frequently, and NA (not applicable).

	Vocal	Social	Facial
0	Moans, whines	Contrary, Unhappy	Furrowed brow
1	Crying	Withdrawn	Eye changes
2	Screaming, yelling	Seeking closeness	Non-smiling
3	Specific word for pain	Inability to distract	Lips tight, quivering
4			Clenching grinding teeth

The child is usually observed for 2 hours and then scored and all scores added. A score of ≥7 indicates pain.

Assessment of pain for cognitively impaired (NCCPC). Activity, Body/Limbs, Physiological, Eating/sleeping

The **Non-communicating Children's Pain Checklist** (NCCPC) is designed for children 3 to 8 who are cognitively impaired but may be used for children recovering from anesthesia (modified version). The checklist contains 7 categories with sublistings that are each scored: 0 (not occurring), 1 occurring occasionally, 2 occurring fairly often, 3 occurring frequently, and NA (not applicable).

Activity	Body/ limbs	Physio-logical	Eating, sleep	Total scores
Still, quiet	Limp	Body shake	Eating less	
Agitated, fidgety	Tense, rigid, spastic	Pallor	Sleep more	
	Pointing to part of body that hurts	Body sweat	Sleep less	
	Guards part of body	Tears		
	Body flinch	Gasps		
	Body shows pain	Holding breath		

The child is usually observed for 2 hours and then scored and all scores added. A score of ≥7 indicates pain.

Preteen/adolescent pain scale

Pain is subjective and may be influenced by the individual's pain sensation threshold (the smallest stimulus that produces the sensation of pain) and tolerance threshold (the maximum degree of pain that a person can tolerate). The most common current pain assessment tool for preteens and adolescents is the 1–10 pain scale.

- 0 = no pain
- 1–2 = mild pain
- 3–5 = moderate pain
- 6–7 = severe pain
- 8–9 = very severe pain
- 10 = excruciating pain

However, assessment also includes information about onset, duration, and intensity. Identifying pain triggers and what relieves it is essential when developing a pain management plan. Children may show very different behaviors when they are in pain: Some may cry and moan with minor pain, and others may seem indifferent even when they are truly suffering. Thus, judging pain by behavior alone can lead to the wrong conclusions.

Family

Identifying primary caregiver

Identifying the primary caregiver is especially important in emergency care of infants and children, as their ability to report is limited and may not be reliable, depending on age. With the diversity of family models, one cannot assume that the mother, father, or person accompanying the child is the primary caregiver. In some cases, custodial arrangements designate one parent as custodial and the other as non-custodial, and they may or may not share legal rights over medical care for the child. In non-traditional families, such as a lesbian couple, laws against same gender marriage may limit legal rights to one parent. Therefore, the nurse should ask who is the primary caregiver in order to glean information about the child and ask who has the legal right to make medical decisions to determine who should sign consent forms and make decisions.

Family functioning and dynamics

Cultural/Lifestyle factors affecting family integration	
Values	Values based on attitudes, ideas, and beliefs often connect family members to common goals. However, these values may be influenced by many external factors, such as education, social norms, and attitudes of peers, other family, and coworkers, so values may change and this may affect family integration.
Roles	In some families, roles are clearly defined by gender and task (homemaker and breadwinner), but the roles blur or are shared in many families, and in some cases the father becomes the primary caregiver while the mother works. Other common roles include peacemaker, nurturer, and social planner. How these roles are perceived and actualized affects the manner in which a child is integrated into the family and cared for.
Decision making	Family power structures vary widely, but in many families power rests with one person who makes ultimate decisions and whose opinions affect other family members. In many traditional cultures (Hispanic, Asian, Middle Eastern) power lies with the father, a grandparent, or other family member. However, in American society, this may vary because of diversity. Power may be shared or rest with the mother or the father.
Socioeconomic	Employment trends, marriage rates, and economic trends all affect family integration. Many people have become unemployed and are unable to support their families, resulting in severe stress, which may be exacerbated by the arrival of a new child or illness. The divorce rate is high, leaving many parents with inadequate funds to support a child. Even if both parents are employed, the cost of living continues to escalate, including the cost of caring for a child.

Nuclear, dual career/dual earner, childless, and extended

Family types	
Nuclear	This husband-wife-children model was once the most common family type but is no longer the norm. In this model, the husband is the provider, and the mother stays home to care for the children, but this makes up only about 7% of current American families.
Dual career/ Dual earner	This model where both parents work is the most common in American society, affecting about 66% of two-parent families. One parent may work more than another or both may work full time. There may be disparities in income that affect family dynamics.
Childless	10–15% have no children because of infertility or choice.
Extended	This may include multigenerational families or shared households with friends, parents, or other relatives. Childcare responsibilities may be shared or primarily assumed by an extended family member, such as a grandparent.
Extended kin network	Two nuclear families live closely together and share goods and services and support each other, including caring for children. This model is common in the Hispanic community.

Single parent and stepparent

Family types	
Single parent	This is one of the fastest growing family models. Usually the mother is the single parent, but in some cases it is the father. The single parent may be widowed, divorced, or separated, but more commonly the person has never married. In cases of divorce or abandonment, the child may have minimal or no contact with one parent, often the father. Single parents often face difficulties in trying to support and care for a child and may suffer economic hardship.
Stepparent	Because of the high rate of divorce, stepparent families are common, and this can result in stress and conflict when a new child enters the picture or a child is ill. There may be jealousy and resentment on the part of siblings and estranged family members. In some cases, families can work together to achieve harmony and provide added support to children.

Binuclear/coparenting, cohabiting, and gay/lesbian

Family types	
Binuclear/ co-parentlng	In this model, children share time between two primarily nuclear families because of joint custody agreements. While this may at times result in conflict, the child benefits from having a continued relationship with both parents.
Cohabiting	Unmarried heterosexual couples live together. The relationships within this model may vary, with some similar to the nuclear family. In some cases, people are in committed relationships and may avoid marriage because of economic or personal reasons. A planned child may strengthen the relationship, but an unplanned child may cause conflict, furthered by the child's illness or injury.
Gay/ Lesbian	In a few states, gays and lesbians can marry, but in most, they cohabit and create families in nontraditional ways. For example, lesbians may use sperm donors. Gay couples often adopt. Children in these families may face social pressures because of their parents' lifestyles, but these children tend to fare as well as those raised in heterosexual households.

Functional coping strategies of families

Some families utilize a number of **functional coping strategies** to deal with stress. These families exhibit resilience in difficult situations. Strategies include:

- Family gathers information, increases organization, discuses issues, and tries to jointly solve problems.
- Family members draw together as a strengthened family unit to deal with stressful situation.
- Family attempts to carry on as normal a routine as possible while making accommodations as needed for a child who is ill. This provides the child with a sense of security.
- Family accepts those things that cannot be changed rather than wasting energy trying to deny or alter reality.
- Family communicates openly and directly, avoiding family secrets and including the child in discussions as appropriate to the child's age.
- Family uses humor to deflect stress.
- Family uses resources outside of the immediate family for support, such as extended family, spiritual advisors, and community agencies.

Dysfunctional coping strategies of families

Some families are not resilient when dealing with stressful situations and exhibit **dysfunctional coping strategies**, which include:

- Family members may resort to substance abuse, such as alcohol and/or drugs, rather than facing problems. This adds to the family dysfunction and negatively affects all members.
- Family may take out frustrations through domestic violence, aimed at the child or other family members. This can include physical, sexual, or mental abuse and can create an environment of fear within the family.
- Family denies problems and refuses to acknowledge that family dynamics have changed, attempting to carry on as usual.
- Family uses threats, aggression, and/or withholding of affection to retain control and maintain the family unit
- Family may blame vulnerable members, such as the child, for the stressful situation, often scapegoating the member that they "blame" rather than dealing with the real problems.

Family support systems and cultural considerations

Cultural considerations:

- **Mexican/Hispanic:** Large extended families may come to visit to support the patient and family, so patients should receive clear explanations about how many visitors are allowed, but some flexibility may be required. In traditional families, the males make decisions, so a woman may wait for the father or other males in the family to make decisions about treatment or care. Families may choose to use folk medicines instead of Western medical care or may combine the two.
- **Middle Eastern:** Families may be accompanied by large extended families that want to be kept informed and whom patients/caregivers consult before making decisions. In Middle Eastern countries, males make decisions, so issues for discussion or decision should be directed to males, while females provide most medical care.
- **Asian:** Families may use healers, cupping, pinching, or applying pressure to injured areas, leaving bruises that may appear as abuse, so the family should be questioned about alternative therapy before making assumptions or passing judgment. In traditional Asian families, males make the decisions.

Patient and Family Care: Managing Technical Skills

IV access and intraosseous (IO) infusion

IV access can be difficult in neonates and infants up until about 2 years. The saphenous vein in the ankle is often accessible, using care to eliminate all air bubbles to prevent air embolism.

Intraosseous (IO) infusion is an alternative to IV access for neonates and pediatric emergencies when rapid access is necessary or when peripheral or vascular access can't be achieved. It is often used in pediatric cardiac arrest. Because yellow marrow replaces red marrow, access in those over 5 is more difficult. Preferred sites include:
0–5: Proximal tibia (preferred).

Older children and adolescents: medial malleolus. The sternum can support higher infusion rates. Other sites include the distal femur, clavicle, humerus, and ileum.

IO infusion is used to administer fluids and anesthesia and to obtain blood samples. Equipment requires a special needle (13–20 gauge) as standard needles may bend. The bone injection gun (BIG) with a loaded spring facilitates insertion. Position is confirmed by aspiration of blood and marrow.

Cardioversion

Cardioversion is a timed electrical stimulation to the heart to convert a tachydysrhythmia (such as atrial fibrillation) to a normal sinus rhythm. During the procedure, the patient is usually sedated and/or anesthetized. Electrodes in the form of gel-covered paddles or pads are positioned on the right subclavicular area and left at 4th and 5th intercostal spaces lateral to nipple. Pads are connected by leads to a computerized ECG and cardiac monitor with a defibrillator. Pediatric paddles are used for children <10 kg. The defibrillator is synchronized with the ECG so that the electrical current is delivered during ventricular depolarization (QRS). The initial dose is 0.5–1 Joule/kg, doubled for subsequent doses if ineffective. The timing must be precise in order to prevent ventricular tachycardia or ventricular fibrillation. Sometimes, drug therapy is used in conjunction with cardioversion; for example, antiarrhythmics may be given before the procedure to slow the heart rate. Complications include dysrhythmias, burns, and injury to myocardium. If ventricular fibrillation occurs, asynchronous shock is used.

Emergency defibrillation

Emergency defibrillation is done to treat acute ventricular fibrillation or ventricular tachycardia in which there is no audible or palpable pulse after 1 minute of CPR. A higher voltage is generally used for defibrillation than is used for cardioversion (initial dose 2 Joules/kg), causing depolarization of myocardial cells, which can then repolarize to regain a normal sinus rhythm. Defibrillation delivers an electrical discharge usually through paddles applied to both sides of the chest. If the first shock and 1 minute of CPR are ineffective, the dose is increased to 4 Joules/kg and 1 minute of CPR, repeated if still ineffective.

After 3 shocks, 1 minute of CPR is followed with epinephrine (0.1mg/kg IV) and another minute of CPR. If still ineffective, other medications (lidocaine 1mg/kg or amiodarone 5mg/kg) may be given followed by CPR. Epinephrine may be readministered every 3–5 minutes with continued CPR.

Normal cardiac rates

Normal cardiac rates can vary widely from one child to another, so it's important to understand the normal range in order to determine if the child has an abnormal pulse. Rates will also vary depending upon whether the child is awake, sleeping, or active. Pulse rate should be taken with a stethoscope, especially for infants and small children the pulse may be difficult to palpate or count accurately manually. Additionally, this allows assessment for heart murmurs.

Newborn infant	At rest: 100–180 Asleep: 80–160 Active/sick: ≤ 220
1–12 weeks	At rest: 100–220 Asleep: 80–200 Active/sick: ≤ 220
3–24 months	At rest: 80–150 Asleep: 70–120 Active/sick: ≤ 200
2–10 years	At rest: 70–110 Asleep: 60–90 Active/sick: ≤ 200
10–adulthood	At rest: 55–90 Asleep: 50–90 Active/sick: ≤ 200

Pacemakers

Children receive **pacemakers** primarily for 3° atrioventricular block, sinus bradycardia, and atrioventricular block that occurs after surgery. Some heart transplant patients may require pacemakers. The parts of the pacemaker include one or two pacing leads (which may elute steroids) that attach to the atrial or ventricular myocardium, or the epicardium in some cases, to sense electrical impulses, leading to an implantable pulse generator (IPG) that contains a lithium battery and microprocessors. In small children, the pacemakers may be placed in the abdomen rather than the shoulder area, which is used for older children. The choice of single- or double-lead pacemakers depends upon the condition of the heart and whether the arrhythmias are atrial, ventricular, or both. The pacemaker is set for the individual and detects electrical impulses, delivers an impulse if necessary, and can be reset noninvasively. Pacemakers prevent the pulse from falling below a certain rate, but also can adjust for activity.

Temporary transvenous pacemakers

The **transvenous pacemaker, a** catheter with a lead at the end, may be used prophylactically or therapeutically on a temporary basis to treat heart block with bradycardia, to improve cardiac output after cardiac surgery, and to decrease ventricular or supraventricular tachycardia by "overdrive" stimulation of contractions. The child is positioned with the head of the bed at 30° to 45° with ECG, pulse oximetry, and noninvasive BP monitoring. The catheter is inserted through the femoral, subclavian, internal or external jugular, or brachial vein, advanced to the right ventricle, and the pacing wire attached to an external pulse generator. The current (in milliamps) is increased until capture occurs. Atrial capture is indicated by a spike immediately preceding a P wave and ventricular capture by a spike immediately preceding the QRS complex. Undersensing and oversensing is evaluated and adjustments to current are made. Current is adjusted to 2 to 3 times threshold value. Rate is age-related, usually starting at 100. Complications are similar to implanted pacemakers and include increased risk of pacemaker syndrome.

Transcutaneous pacing

Transcutaneous pacing is used temporarily to treat bradydysrhythmia that doesn't respond to medications (atropine) and results in hemodynamic instability. Generally, an arterial line is placed, pulse oximetry monitored, and the patient provided oxygen and sedation before pacing. The placement of pacing pads (large self-adhesive pads) and ECG leads varies somewhat according to the type of equipment, but the anterior-anterior position for pacing pads is usually used with infants and young children while the anterior-posterior is used for obese or older children. Lead wires attach the pads to the monitor. The rate of pacing is usually started at 100 for children, but this setting is age related. Current (milliamps) is increased slowly until capture occurs—a spiking followed by QRS complex, then the current is adjusted to 1.5 times the point of capture. Both demand and fixed modes are available, but demand mode is preferred. Patients may require analgesia, especially if a higher current setting is needed, as they may experience burning/tingling. Pads are changed every 8 hours.

Pacemaker problems

Problems associated with pacemakers	
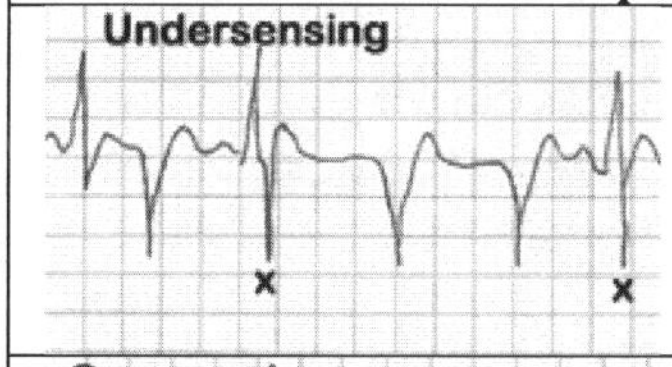	**Undersensing:** The sensitivity is too low to detect cardiac depolarizations and triggers unneeded contractions, competing with patient's native rhythm. This may be related to dislodging of lead, incorrect positioning of lead, or low-amplitude cardiac signal.
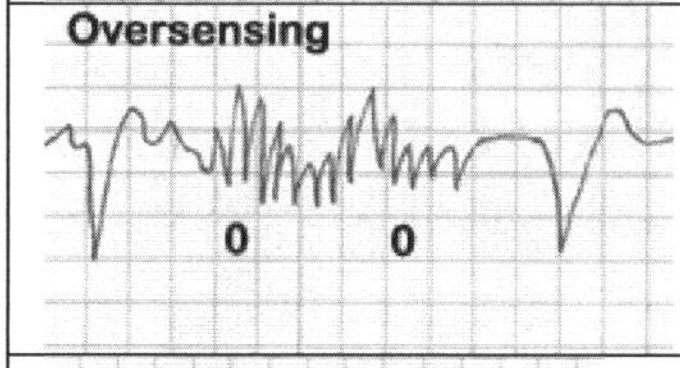	**Oversensing:** The sensitivity is too high and misinterprets artifacts (such as muscle contractions) and non-depolarization events as contractions and fails to trigger, resulting in decreased cardiac output because of interruption in contractions. This may result from damage or disconnection of lead.
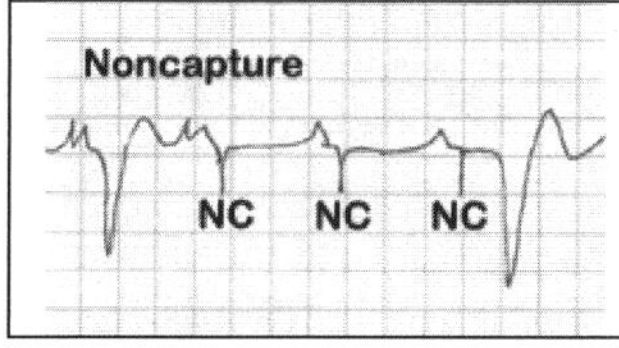	**Noncapture:** The pacemaker does not trigger contractions. This may be related to settings, lead disconnection, low battery, or metabolic changes

Peripheral intravenous access

Peripheral intravenous access in children can be quite difficult, especially in young (≤3) or seriously ill or injured children, with most children requiring 2 or more punctures before a line is established. Veins in the hands and feet are often used for small children. If time permits, a local or topical anesthetic should be used. Common equipment includes over-the-needle catheters or butterfly needles. All IV tubing and solutions should be flushed and prepared before venipuncture. Steps include:

- Provide caregiver and child (age-appropriate) explanation of procedure and purpose.
- Use comfort positioning (such as hug hold) and distractions for young children.
- Use various methods to help locate veins: warm area, apply blood pressure cuff or tourniquet, apply topical nitroglycerin, tap vein, or use transillumination or ultrasound.
- Cleanse skin according to protocol in a circular motion (inside to outward) with povidone iodine or 70% alcohol and allow to air dry.
- Insert needle/catheter, usually with bevel up and at 20–30° angle to skin.
- Attach appropriate tubing.

Peripherally inserted central catheters (PICC lines)

Peripherally inserted central catheters (PICC) are used for extended intravenous access or those with limited access. Insertion sites include the scalp, axilla, brachial cephalic saphenous and basilic veins.

- Measure the catheter insertion length:
- Hand/arm: Insertion site to axilla and to 1 cm above nipple line.
- Scalp: Insertion site to 1 cm above nipple line.
- Leg: Insertion site to 1 cm above umbilicus.
- Apply topical (EMLA) or local anesthetic for 30 minutes and maintain the child's temperature at 36°–37°C.
- Restrain an infant's limbs to prevent contamination of sterile field.

If catheter is inserted in the hand or arm, turn the child's head toward insertion site to partially occlude the jugular vein and reduce risk of catheter entering the jugular.

After insertion above the waist, the catheter should be in the superior vena cava above the right atrium. PICC lines in lower extremities should lie in the inferior vena cava below the right atrium. AP and lateral radiographs, ultrasound, or echocardiogram verify correct placement.

Central venous access devices

Central venous catheters can be inserted into the subclavian, femoral, or internal jugular veins for those who need long-term IV access or who cannot have a peripheral IV. The subclavian is most commonly used for children, but the femoral access site may be used in emergencies or during CPR. Position is verified by radiograph. Tunneled CVCs are inserted surgically under general or local anesthesia. Tunneling increases the life of the catheter and reduces incidence of infection. In emergent situations, non-tunneled catheters are used. Some catheters have multiple lumens. Indications of complications include erythema, tenderness, exudate, fever (≥38° C/100.5° F), edema, and leakage around catheter. Each lumen is usually flushed with heparinized saline (100 U/mL) (3–10 mL) daily or weekly, depending on the type of catheter. Injection caps are changed every 5–7 days.

Implanted central venous infusion ports

Implanted central venous infusion ports, such as PORT-A-CATH®, comprise a self-sealing injection port and an attached venous catheter. The port is surgically inserted under the skin, often in the infraclavicular fossa, and the catheter fed into the right atrium. Position is verified by radiograph. Special 20–22 gauge non-coring Huber needles are used to access the port through the skin. The port must be checked for patency before administering any medications, blood, or fluids by aspirating blood return. For infusions, 90° needles are inserted perpendicularly to the port. Before withdrawing the needle, the tubing must be clamped and positive pressure applied to prevent reflux. The port should be flushed with 3–6 mL NS before and after administration of medications. The port must be flushed with heparinized saline (100 U/mL) (3–5 mL) after every use or at least one time monthly if not being used.

Cardiac output, stroke volume, and heart rate

In order to understand the hemodynamics of infants and children, it's important to understand the **relationship among cardiac output, heart rate, and stroke volume** as the child grows and cardiac size increases.

Age	CO	SV	HR
Newborn	800 mL/ min	5 mL	145
6 months	1000–1600 mL/min	10 mL	120
12 months	1400 mL/min	13 mL	115
4 years	2300 mL/min	26 mL	105
8 years	3500 mL/min	42 mL	83
10 years	4000 mL/min	50 mL	75
15 years (adult levels)	5000 to 6000 mL/min	85 mL	70

Hemodynamic monitoring and mixed venous gases/SvO2

Mixed venous gases (MVG), especially venous oxygen saturation (SvO2), are monitored for indications of respiratory failure, reduced oxygenation, anemia, and changes in cardiac output. Mixed venous gas refers to venous blood that has returned to the heart from the superior and inferior vena cava and the coronary sinus. Obtaining a sample from the right atrium may reflect primarily blood from the superior vena cava, which usually has a lower saturation (70%) than the blood from the inferior vena cava (80%) or the coronary sinus (56%). The blood in the right ventricle and pulmonary artery is completed "mixed" and the saturation averaged. MVG is usually measured by sampling through a pulmonary artery catheter. Normal values:

- **PCO_2:** 41–51 mm Hg (pulmonary venous carbon dioxide pressure)
- **PvO_2:** 35–49 mm Hg (pulmonary venous oxygen pressure)
- **SvO_2:** 60–80% (pulmonary venous oxygen saturation.

If there is a decrease in SvO_2, then the oxygenation is not sufficient for tissue needs.

Left atrial pressure

Left atrial pressure may be monitored in the postsurgical period by way of a catheter inserted during surgery into the left atrium from the right superior pulmonary vein or through the left atrial appendage. Oxygen saturation of blood in the left atrium should be 100%. Left atrial pressures:

- **Normal values:** 1–2 mm Hg higher than right atrial pressure (4–12 mg Hg). Pressure above 12–14 postsurgically is cause for concern.
- **Increased** pressure may indicate an increase in end-diastolic pressure of the left ventricle, a decrease in function, hypertrophy, heart failure, or an increase in left ventricular afterload. An increase may also indicate mitral valve stenosis, backflow, or thrombus obstruction, a significant right to left shunt, excessive intravascular volume, tachycardia with arrhythmias, or cardiac tamponade.
- **Decreased** pressure may indicate a decrease in intravascular fluid or insufficient preload.

Pulmonary artery pressure and pulmonary artery/capillary wedge pressure

- **Pulmonary artery pressure (PAP)** is measured by a catheter usually fed through the right ventricle to the main pulmonary artery, measuring systolic, diastolic, and mean pressures, with the patient in supine position ≤45° elevation.
- **Normal values:** 10–20 mg Hg (mean 15 mm Hg). Postoperative rates should be <25 mm Hg. PAP is usually about 25–34% the systemic blood pressure rate. Oxygen saturation is usually about 80%. **Increased** pressure may indicate pulmonary obstruction or embolus, left to right shunt, left ventricular failure, pulmonary hypertension, or mitral stenosis, pneumothorax, lung/alveolar hypoplasia, hyperviscosity of blood, or increased left atrial pressure.
- **Decreased** pressure may indicate a decrease in intravascular volume or cardiac output, or obstruction of pulmonary blood flow.

The catheter may have a balloon that can be inflated in the pulmonary artery to provide a measurement of **pulmonary artery/capillary wedge pressure (PAWP/PCWP)** to evaluate pulmonary hypertension, left ventricular failure, and mitral stenosis.
Normal values: 4–12 mm Hg. **Increased pressure** may indicate left ventricular failure, mitral insufficiency or mitral stenosis.

Central venous/right atrial pressure

Central venous pressure (CVP) (right atrial), the pressure in the right atrium or vena cava, is used to assess function of the right ventricles, preload, and flow of venous blood to the heart. The CVP catheter may be placed during surgery or inserted via the internal jugular (usually under ultrasound) or external jugular, subclavian (higher risk of pneumothorax), or femoral vein (higher risk of infection). Heparin flush is used to prevent clotting. Normal pressure ranges from 1–7 mm Hg in children but may be elevated after surgery. Incorrect catheter placement or malfunctioning can affect readings:

- **Increased CVP** is related to overload of intravascular volume caused by decreased function, hypertrophy, or failure of the right ventricle; increased right ventricular afterload, tricuspid valve stenosis, regurgitation, or thrombus obstruction; or shunt from left ventricle to right atrium. It can also be caused by arrhythmias or cardiac tamponade.
- **Decreased CVP** is related to low intravascular volume, decreased preload, or vasodilation.

Intraarterial blood pressure monitoring/MAP

Intraarterial blood pressure monitoring is done for systolic, diastolic, and **mean arterial pressure (MAP)** for conditions that decrease cardiac output, tissue perfusion, or fluid volume. A catheter is inserted into an artery, such as the radial, dorsalis pedis, femoral, or axillary, percutaneously or through a cut-down. Before catheter insertion, collateral circulation must be assessed by Doppler or the Allen test (used for the hand). In the Allen test, both the radial and ulnar artery are compressed and the patient is asked to clench the hand repeatedly until it blanches, and then one artery is released, and the tissue on that side should flush. Then the test is repeated again, releasing the other artery. The MAP is most commonly used to evaluate perfusion as it shows pressure throughout the cardiac cycle. Systole is one-third and diastole two-thirds of the normal cardiac cycle. The MAP for a blood pressure of 100/60 (normal range 70–100 mm Hg with 60 the critical level):
[(Diastole x 2) + (Systole x 1)] / 3 = MAP

For example: (60 x 2 = 120) + (100) = 220/3 = MAP of 73.3.

Perfusion pressure and pulse pressure

The **perfusion pressure** (measured by the MAP) that is necessary may vary with different conditions and circumstances. The **pulse pressure** is the difference between systolic and diastolic pressures, and this can be an important indicator. For example, with a decrease in cardiac output, vasoconstriction takes place in the body's attempt to maintain the blood pressure. In this case, the MAP may remain unchanged, but the pulse pressure narrows. Necessary values for MAP include:

- >60 mm Hg to perfuse coronary arteries
- 70–90 mm Hg to perfuse the brain and other organs, such as the kidneys, and to maintain cardiac patients and decrease the workload of the left ventricle
- 90–110 to increase cerebral perfusion after neurosurgical procedures, such as carotid endarterectomy

Patients should be assessed for changes in pulse pressure that may be precipitated by medications, such as diuretics that alter fluid volume.

Incision and drainage

Incision and drainage is generally the treatment of choice for abscesses, which can occur in almost any part of the body, especially those affected by infection or trauma. Typical signs and symptoms associated with abscess include erythema, swelling, pain, and fluctuation as the abscess comes to a head; however, fluctuation may be a late sign, and early intervention may prevent further tissue damage or development of fistulae. Incision and drainage is usually done with local anesthetic, but further sedation may be necessary, depending on the age of the child. To differentiate an abscess from other problems, such as a hematoma, a small amount of fluid may be aspirated with a 22- to 23-gauge needle prior to incision. In many cases, a drain or packing may be left in place to ensure the abscess does not recur. Common abscesses in children include perianal abscess, peritonsillar abscess, retropharyngeal, submandibular, axillary, and cervical.

Dressing products

There is a wide variety of **dressing products**, and there is not one dressing that can suffice for all wounds. Dressings should be chosen according to the type of wound and the function of the dressing. A series of different types of dressings may be used during the healing process. There are 3 main types of dressings to consider when determining which will be the most effective for a particular type of wound:
Traditional topical dressings that are used primarily to cover the wound, such as gauze and tulle.
Interactive dressings, such as polymeric films, are generally transparent so that the wound can be observed and are permeable to water vapor and oxygen but provide an effective barrier for microorganisms, such as hyaluronic acid, hydrogels and foam dressings.

Bioactive dressings provide substances that directly promote wound healing, such as hydrocolloids, alginates, collagens, and chitosan.

Primary, secondary, and tertiary healing

- **Primary healing** (healing by first intention) involves a wound that is surgically closed by suturing, flaps, or split- or full-thickness grafts to completely cover the wound. Primary healing is the most common approach used for surgeries or repair of wounds or lacerations, especially when the wound is essentially "clean."
- **Secondary healing** (healing by second intention) involves leaving the wound open and allowing it to close through granulation and epithelialization. Debridement of the wound is done to prepare the wound bed for healing. This approach may be used with contaminated "dirty" or infected wounds to prevent abscess formation and allow the wound to drain.
- **Tertiary healing** (healing by third intention) is also sometimes called delayed primary closure because it involves first debriding the wound and allowing it to begin healing while open and then later closing the wound through suturing or grafts. This approach is common with wounds that are contaminated, such as severe animal bites, or wounds related to mixed trauma.

Primary phases of wound healing

There are 4 primary phases of wound healing:

- **Hemostasis** takes place within the first few minutes after injury and bleeding when the platelets begin to seal off the vessels and secrete substances that cause vasoconstriction. Thrombin is produced to stimulate the clotting mechanism, forming a fibrin mesh.
- **Inflammation (lag or exudative)** occurs over days 1–4. During this phase, there is erythema and edema along with pain as the blood vessels release plasma and neutrophils or polymorphonucleocytes to begin phagocytosis to remove debris and prevent infection.
- **Proliferation/granulation (fibroblastic)** occurs over days 5–20. During this phase, fibroblasts produce collagen to provide support, and granulation tissue starts to form. Epithelization occurs as does contracture of the wound.
- **Maturation (differentiation, remodeling or plateau)** occurs after day 21 for an indeterminate duration. The fibroblasts leave the wound and the collagen tightens to reduce scarring. The tissue gains tensile strength. This stage can take up to 2 years, and the wound can break down easily again during this phase.

Partial-thickness and full-thickness wounds and healing

Partial-thickness wounds involve only the epidermis and the upper parts of the dermis, so the underlying structures that repair skin and provide nutrients, such as the vasculature, and protection, such as the glands, remain intact. Bleeding activates hemostasis and provides a temporary bacterial barrier. Coagulation occurs and fibrin is formed with the clot sealing disrupted vessels. This is followed by fibrinolysis, during which the clot breaks down and repair begins with the inflammatory stage. Healing phases progress and wounds usually heal within about 2 weeks.

Full-thickness wounds involve the loss of the epidermis and dermis and may also involve loss of underlying tissues, through the fascia, muscle, and to the bone. Full-thickness wounds may be acute or chronic and heal by primary or secondary intention. Those healing by secondary intention are usually surgical wounds that have dehisced or those resulting from underlying morbidities that interfere with normal healing. Bleeding and hemostasis do not occur with healing by secondary intention, compromising the healing process.

Monitoring of intracranial pressure

Monitoring of intracranial pressure in pediatric patients is of special importance because of the danger of herniation with increased pressure. Studies indicate that intracranial pressure requires treatment if ≥20 mm Hg, although some authorities believe that infants and young children may need treatment at lower pressures. Monitoring of intracranial pressure can be done in a number of ways:

- Intraventricular catheter attached to a transducer to record pressure (most accurate)
- Subarachnoid bolt
- Epidural or subdural catheter
- Fiberoptic transducer-tipped catheter placed in the ventricular or subdural space
- External anterior fontanel monitor

CSF may be drained continuously or intermittently and must be monitored hourly for amount, color, and character. For ICP measurement, the patient's head must be elevated to 30° to 45° and the transducer leveled to the outer canthus of the eye. Normal ICP values (manometer):

- Infant: 1.5 to 6 mm Hg
- Young child: 3 to 7 mm Hg
- Older child: 2 to 7 mm Hg
- 18 years: 0 to 15 mm Hg

Monroe-Kellie hypothesis

The **Monroe-Kellie hypothesis** states that to maintain a normal intracranial pressure (ICP), a change in volume in one compartment must be compensated by a reciprocal change in volume in another compartment. The three brain compartments are brain tissue, cerebrospinal fluid (CSF), and blood. The CSF and blood can change more easily to accommodate changes in pressure than tissue, so medical intervention focuses on cerebral blood flow and drainage. Symptoms include:

- **Infants:** Bulging fontanels without normal pulsations, distention of scalp veins, and increased head circumference. Infants may be irritable with high-pitched cries and poor feeding.
- **Children:** Headache, vomiting without associated nausea, double and blurred vision, seizures. Behavioral and personality changes may occur, increased lethargy, memory loss, and inability to follow directions.
- **Late signs:** Decreased level of consciousness, motor response, and response to painful stimuli. Pupil size and reactivity change, decerebrate or decorticate posturing, respiratory depression with Cheyne-Stokes and papilledema. Cushing's triad:
    - Increased systolic pressure with widened pulse pressure
    - Bradycardia in response to increased pressure
    - Decreased respirations

Chest tubes

Chest tubes are inserted to treat pneumothorax, hemothorax, pleural effusion, penetrating thoracic trauma, and pleural empyema. A chest tube may be inserted during thoracic surgery or for instillation of medications (such as fibrinolytic agents). Chest tube sizes vary with the age and size of the child.

- 0–12 months: 10 to 12 F

- 1–3 years: 16 to 20 F
- 6 years: 20 to 28 F
- 10 years: 28 to 32 F
- 13+ years: 32 to 42 F

Child is positioned supine with arm on affected side elevated and immobilized and thorax slightly rotated to expose insertion site. Sedation and local anesthetic are administered as indicated. Insertion sites include:

- 4th or 5th intercostal space, midaxillary line
- 2nd intercostal space, midclavicular line

Once chest tube is in place, it is attached to a closed drainage system. Chest x-ray confirms proper placement of chest tube. Complications include bleeding (increased drainage), clotting of tube (decreased drainage), air leaks, and infection.

Closed drainage systems for chest tubes

Chest tubes with a closed drainage system are usually left in place after thoracic surgery or pneumothorax to drain air or fluid.
Water seal (wet suction): 3-chambered system with one chamber for collection, the middle for water seal, and the third for wet suction control. Sterile fluid must be instilled into the middle and suction chambers. The system contains both positive and negative pressure release valves and bubbles intermittently if functioning properly. Chambers must be in upright position.

Water seal (dry suction): Similar 3-chambered system but sterile fluid must be instilled to 2 cm level in water seal chamber only. A regulator controls suction, and an indicator shows if suction pressure is correct. Dry suction has positive and negative release values and chambers must be in upright position.

Dry suction (one-way valve): 2-chambered system with mechanical valve allows air to leave chest but not enter. This system has a collection chamber and a dry suction control chamber, requires no fluid instillation, and need not be in upright position, so it is useful for ambulatory children.

Nasopharyngeal wash

Nasopharyngeal wash obtains a diagnostic specimen for diagnosis of influenzae A and B, RSV, adenovirus, and parainfluenzae types I, II, and III. Contraindications include thrombocytopenia (<20,000), respiratory distress (oximetry ≤90%), epistaxis, and lesions or nasopharyngeal trauma. Procedure:

- Don personal protective equipment and exam gloves.
- Fill two 3–5 mL syringes with 1–4 mL of normal saline (nonbacteriostatic), depending on patient's age and size. Attach soft catheter (6 Fr for neonate, 8 Fr for infants and toddlers, and 10 Fr for school-age children).
- Estimate the length of catheter necessary to reach the nasopharynx (usually about 1.5 to 2 inches).
- Tilt the patient's head into sniff position and hold one nostril closed while inserting NS into the other nostril. Do not apply lubricant to the catheter.
- Gently aspirate fluid while removing the catheter.
- Inject aspirant into sterile container.

- Repeat procedure with the other nostril.

Traction splinting

Traction splints are applied for fractures of long bones, such as midshaft fractures of the femur, in order to reduce pain and prevent further damage to tissue and vasculature. Procedures may vary slightly with different types of traction splints. Two people are usually required.

- Begin by fitting the splint to the uninjured limb so that it can be adjusted to fit properly.
- Assess circulation including pedal pulses, toe movement, and sensation while a partner manually stabilizes the femur.
- Apply manual traction by holding above the ankle and below the knee (only if no lower leg injury is suspected).
- Slide the splint below the limb.
- Secure the splint with straps, usually 2 above knee and two below, being careful to avoid area of fracture and attaching the ischial strap first.
- Apply ankle strap.
- Apply traction hook to ankle strap.
- Adjust traction until it takes over for manual traction.
- Reassess pain level, pedal pulses, toe movement, and sensation.

For transport, the patient is placed on a long board with the splint secured to the board.

Collecting urine specimens

Collecting urine specimens	
Infant	Cleanse perineal area and apply sterile urine collection bag according to manufacturer's guidelines.
Child	**Standard:** Use a collection hat in toilet or provide an older child with a specimen cup, urinal, or bedpan. **Midstream:** Explain in detail about cleansing and urinating procedures. Assist or ask a parent to assist a younger child. **Timed specimen:** Obtain proper storage bottle with chemical additive and ensure that everyone caring for the child knows the duration of the timed specimen (12 hours, 24 hours) and post a sign. Label the collection bottle and ensure it is refrigerated or placed on ice if necessary. Provide a bedpan, urinal, specimen hat, or potty chair as appropriate to obtain specimen. **Indwelling catheter:** Clamp for 30 minutes. Use 3 mL syringe for culture and 20 mL syringe for urinalysis. Cleanse port or self-sealing catheter directly above connecting tube and allow to dry. Insert needle (1 inch 21 gauge) into port/catheter at 45° angle and withdraw urine. Inject urine into sterile specimen container.

Capillary blood sampling

Neonatal **capillary blood sampling** is a common procedure used to acquire small samples of blood for testing of glucose and drug levels, blood gases, electrolytes, urea, blood counts, and other screening tests. If done incorrectly, it can cause pain, trauma, and nerve damage. The lancet should be ≤2.4 mm deep. The baby should be supine.

- Grasp the foot with one hand holding the ankle with the thumb and index finger and supporting the leg with the other fingers.
- Cleanse the infant's heel (bottom, lateral aspect only to avoid nerves in the middle of the foot) thoroughly with water (not alcohol) and air-dry.

- Hold the skin of the heel tight until after the puncture, and then relax it and lightly compress the heel to express a drop of blood, which is collected in a capillary tube. Relaxing the pressure and then compressing again will "milk" additional drops.
- Apply pressure to the puncture site until bleeding stops and then apply a dressing.

Nasogastric and orogastric enteral feeding tubes

Nasogastric/orogastric enteral feeding tubes can be inserted quickly and nonsurgically but are usually reserved for short-term (<3 months) enteral feedings. A weighted or non-weighted catheter (5 to 8 Fr) is used. The length of insertion can be calculated using age-related height-based measurement or measuring the distance from the nose tip to earlobe and earlobe to the midpoint between the xiphoid process and the umbilicus.

- Mark the insertion length on the tube.
- Explain the procedure in age-appropriate terms.
- Check nares for patency, assess gag reflex, and note any contraindications (such as basal skull fracture with NG tubes).
- Secure child in supine position (swaddling, holding) with head elevated to 30°–45°.
- Lubricate tube or dip in water for pre-lubricated tubes.
- Insert the tube into the mouth or nostril aiming posteriorly and inferiorly.
- When the NG/OG tube is in the pharynx, instruct the child to swallow or stimulate swallowing with use of pacifier.
- Insert to marking on tube and temporarily secure.
- Verify placement with radiograph.

Gastrointestinal feeding tubes placement

- **Surgical placement:** There are both open and laparoscopic surgical techniques for placing tubes to the stomach or jejunum. The three most common methods are the Janeway, the Stamm, and the Witzel techniques.
- **Endoscopic placement:** Percutaneous endoscopic gastrostomy (PEG) involves intubation of the esophagus with the endoscope and insertion of a sheathed needle with a guidewire through the abdomen and stomach wall so that a catheter can be fed down the esophagus, snared, and pulled out through the opening where the needle was inserted and secured. Similar endoscopic procedures can be done in the jejunum.
- **Radiologic placement:** Through fluoroscopy, ultrasound and/or CT, a gastrostomy tube is inserted through the epigastrium and secured with a balloon and external bumper or disk. Insertion into the jejunum is done in a similar manner through the duodenum into the jejunum. A gastrojejunostomy tube, which both drains the stomach and feeds the jejunum, is another procedure.

Nutritional assessment for enteral feedings

Caloric and nutritional needs for enteral feedings are assessed according to the age of the child, size, and stress factors. Breast milk is the optimal nutrition for infants. Feedings may be adjusted because of needs associated with diseases; for example, children with HF may require fluid restriction. Formula usually contains 24–30 calories per ounce. Caloric requirements are based on the RDA and resting energy expenditure (REE), the calories needed for a child at rest.

Age	RDA: Kcal/kg/d	REE: Kcal/kg/d	Protein: g/kg/d
6 -12 months	90 to 108	55	2 to 2.5
1 to 3 years	85 to 102	50 to 57	1.2 to 3
4 to 6 years	70 to 90	45 to 48	1.1 to 3
7 to 10 years	60 to 70	40	1.0 to 3
11 to 13 years	45 to 55	28 to 32	1.0 to 2.5
14 to 18 years	36 to 45	25 to 27	0.8 to 1.2

Total energy expenditure (TEE) is calculated by multiplying the REE by stress factors:

Maintenance: 0.2
Activity: 0.1 to 0.25
Fever: 0.13 per degree >38°C
Burns: 0.5 to 1
Simple trauma: 0.2
Sepsis/major trauma: 0.4 to 1.5
Ventilation/sedation: 1.2 to 1.3
Growth: 0.5

Preventing displacement of enteral feeding tubes

The displacement of an enteral feeding tube is usually the result of inadequate stabilization. Foley catheters must be marked where they exit the stoma to check for migration. Gastrostomy tubes with an internal balloon or mushroom tip, measured markings, and an external disk are easier to stabilize, but internal device should be checked daily by gently pulling until resistance is felt. External stabilizing devices can be applied to the skin to hold the tube in place. The tube may also be taped to the abdomen or secured with a binder. Sometimes surgeons suture the tube in place, especially those with no balloon, such as jejunostomy tubes, which can become easily dislodged. A solid skin barrier with the tube fed through an anchored baby nipple is an inexpensive stabilizer. Position and length of tube should be carefully documented. Balloon volume should be checked weekly to insure there are no leaks. Skin beneath disks/bumpers should be checked frequently.

Preventing and treating occlusion of enteral feeding tubes

Prevention of occlusion of enteral feeding tubes involves proper administration of medications and feedings, and maintaining a regular schedule of flushing. Tubes should be flushed with 5–30 ml of water (depending on age and size of child) at least every 4 hours as well as before and after feedings and administration of medications. Medications should be in liquid form or crushed completely and enteric-coated or delayed release preparations should be avoided. Feeding solutions should be liquid consistency. Child should be positioned with head elevated for feedings.

Flushing of occluded tube involves first checking for kinks or obvious problems, attaching a 20–30 ml syringe and aspirating fluid. Then, 5–10 ml of water or carbonated beverage (ginger ale, cola) can be slowly instilled (over about a minute) and aspirated a number of times to try to loosen occlusion. After clamping for 10–15 minutes, the flushing procedure can be repeated with warm water/carbonated beverage. If the water or carbonated beverage fails, a multi-enzyme cocktail or Pancrease and sodium bicarbonate solution may succeed. If all flushing fails, the physician should be notified.

Chemical or biological decontamination

The nurse must avoid self-contamination during decontamination procedures for **chemical or biological decontamination.** Staff members must wear appropriate protective gear during procedures that place them at risk.

- **Level A:** (highest level) Fully encapsulating suit, boots, inner gloves, outer gloves, and self-contained breathing apparatus with faceplate extending from hair to chin and tank for air.
- **Level B:** Similar to level A except that the suit is hooded rather than fully encapsulating.
- **Level C:** Same as level B except that a canister filter or HEPA filter (especially valuable with biological agents) is used with room air instead of a self-contained breathing apparatus. This level is appropriate only if oxygen levels are adequate and if the hazardous material is known and does not require level A or B protection.

Confirming correct placement of endotracheal tubes

There are a number of methods to confirm correct placement of **endotracheal tubes**. Clinical assessment alone is not adequate.

- **Capnometry** utilizes an end-tidal CO_2 ($ETCO_2$) detector that measures the concentration of CO_2 in expired air, usually through pH-sensitive paper that changes color (commonly purple to yellow). The capnometer is attached to the ETT with a bag-valve-mask (BVM) ventilator attached. The child is provided 6 ventilations and the CO_2 concentration checked.
- **Capnography** is attached to the ETT and provides a waveform graph, showing the varying concentrations of CO_2 in real time throughout each ventilation (with increased CO_2 on expiration) and can indicate changes in respiratory status.
- **Esophageal detection devices** fit over the end of the ETT so that a large syringe can be used to attempt to aspirate. If the ETT is in the esophagus, the walls collapse on aspiration and resistance occurs whereas the syringe fills with air if the ETT is in the trachea. A self-inflating bulb (Ellick® device) may also be used.

Ventilator management

There are many types of ventilators now in use, and the specific directions for use of each type must be followed carefully, but there are general principles that apply to all **ventilator management.** The following should be monitored:

- **Type of ventilation:** volume-cycled, pressure-cycled, negative-pressure, HFJV, HFOV, CPAP, Bi-PAP.
- **Control mode:** controlled ventilation, assisted ventilation, synchronized intermittent mandatory (allows spontaneous breaths between ventilator controlled inhalation/exhalation), positive end expiratory pressure (PEEP) (positive pressure at end of expiration), CPAP, Bi-PAP.
- **Tidal volume** (TV) range should be set in relation to respiratory rate.
- **Inspiratory-expiratory ratio** (I:E) usually ranges from 1:2–1:5, but may vary.
- **Respiratory rate** will depend upon TV and $PaCO_2$ target.
- **Fraction of inspired oxygen** (FiO_2) (percentage of oxygen in the inspired air), ranging from 21–100%, usually maintained <40% to avoid toxicity.
- **Sensitivity** determines the effort needed to trigger inspiration.
- **Pressure** controls the pressure exerted in delivering TV.
- **Rate of flow** controls the L/min speed of TV.

Positive pressure ventilators

Positive pressure ventilators assist respiration by applying pressure directly to the airway, inflating the lungs, forcing expansion of the alveoli, and facilitating gas exchange. Generally, endotracheal intubation or tracheostomy is necessary to maintain positive pressure ventilation for extended periods. There are 3 basic kinds of positive pressure ventilators:

- **Pressure cycled:** This type of ventilation is usually used for short-term treatment in adolescents or adults. The IPPB machine is the most common type. This delivers a flow of air to a preset pressure and then cycles off. Airway resistance or changes in compliance can affect volume of air and may compromise ventilation.
- **Time cycled:** This type of ventilation regulates the volume of air the patient receives by controlling the length of inspiration and the flow rate.
- **Volume cycled:** This type of ventilation provides a preset flow of pressurized air during inspiration and then cycles off and allows passive expiration, providing a fairly consistent volume of air.

Noninvasive positive pressure ventilators

Noninvasive positive pressure ventilators provide air through a tight-fitting nasal or face mask, usually pressure cycled, avoiding the need for intubation and reducing the danger of hospital-acquired infection and mortality rates. It can be used for acute respiratory failure and pulmonary edema. There are 2 types of noninvasive positive pressure ventilators:

- **CPAP (Continuous positive airway pressure)** provides a steady stream of pressurized air throughout both inspiration and expiration. CPAP improves breathing by decreasing preload and afterload for children with congestive heart failure. It reduces the effort required for breathing and improves compliance of the lung.
- **Bi-PAP (Bi-level positive airway pressure)** provides a steady stream of pressurized air like CPAP but it senses inspiratory effort and increases pressure during inspiration. Bi-PAP pressures for inspiration and expiration can be set independently. Machines can be programmed with a backup rate to ensure a set number of respirations per minute.

Moving an injured child from a child safety seat

Procedures for **moving an injured child from a child safety seat** may vary depending on the child's condition and whether the child safety seat is inside a motor vehicle involved in an accident or the child was transported to the ED in the seat. The first step is to carefully note and later document the child's position in the seat and whether the harness is properly secured with the fastener over the sternum. If the harness is too loose, the child is at increased risk of fractures and/or internal injuries. If the fastener is too low, the risk of rib fractures increases. A cervical collar should be placed about the child's neck before moving. The harness should be cut away from the child, to avoid unnecessary movement, unless the child is moving freely. If possible, a small backboard should be slipped behind the child before the child is lifted from the seat; otherwise, the child should be well-supported and moved to a pediatric board placed beside the seat and the child's head secured in neutral position.

Spinal immobilization

Infants and children with multiple trauma or suspected spinal trauma should be placed in a cervical collar and secured to a backboard for **spinal immobilization**. Indications of spinal trauma include tenderness over spinous processes and motor and/or sensory deficits. Pediatric boards should be used because they allow for the larger head size of the child, and placing the child on an adult board may result in airway occlusion as the head is forced forward. The child should be moved onto the board with as little movement as possible. If the child is lying in supine position, the child should be lifted straight up and placed on the board rather than rolled onto the board. However, if the child is lying in prone position, the child should be rolled directly onto the board. For motorcycle accidents, spinal mobilization must be maintained during removal of the helmet. For football accidents, shoulder pads and helmet should be left in place initially but the facemask removed.

Hold positions for procedures

Pediatric comfort holding positions	
Hug hold	Position an infant or small child facing the caregiver and straddling the caregiver's legs with the caregiver's arms securely hugging the child. Another person should distract the child or secure free arm(s). Good position for injections and venipuncture.
Side sitting	Similar to hug hold with the child facing the caregiver but legs to the side. Good position for older children who want less confinement.
Bracing	Child is held in supine position in the caregiver's arms and braced against the chest or shoulder to prevent movement of the head. Good position for insertion of NG tubes or examination/treatment of mouth or other parts of face.
Sitting	Child sits forward or sideways on caregiver's lap with caregiver's arms around child. Good position for children who want to watch or don't want to be more confined.
Supine	Child lies on table with caregiver behind the child so the child's head lies on the caregiver's lap while the caregiver holds the child or provides distraction.

Administration of 12-lead ECG

The **electrocardiogram** provides a graphic representation of the electrical activity of the heart. It is indicated for chest pain, dyspnea, syncope, acute coronary syndrome, pulmonary embolism, and possible MI. The standard 12-lead ECG gives a picture of electrical activity from 12 perspectives through placement of 10 body leads:

- 4 limb leads are placed distally on the wrists and ankles (but may be placed more proximally if necessary),

Precordial leads:

- V1: right sternal border at 4th intercostal space
- V2: left sternal border at 4th intercostal space
- V3: Midway between V2 and V4
- V4: Left midclavicular line at 5th intercostal space
- V5: Horizontal to V4 at left anterior axillary line
- V6: Horizontal to V5 at left midaxillary line

In some cases, additional leads may be used: Right-sided leads are placed on the right in a mirror image of the left leads, usually to diagnose right ventricular infarction through ST elevation.

Airway devices

Airways are used to establish a patent airway and facilitate respirations.

- **Oropharyngeal** is a plastic airway curves over the tongue and creates space between the mouth and the posterior pharynx. It is used for anesthetized or unconscious children to keep tongue and epiglottis from blocking the airway.
- **Nasopharyngeal** (trumpet) is a smaller flexible airway is more commonly used in conscious children and is inserted through one nostril, extending to the nasopharynx.
- **Tracheostomy tubes**-Tracheostomy may be utilized for mechanical ventilation. Tubes are inserted into the opening to provide a conduit and maintain the opening. Tracheostomy tubes are usually silastic or plastic, most lacking an inner cannula because they are non-

adherent. The tube is secured with ties around the neck. Because the air entering the lungs through the tracheostomy bypasses the warming and moistening affects of the upper airway, air is humidified through a room humidifier or through delivery of humidified air through a special mask or mechanical ventilation.

- **The laryngeal-mask airway** (LMA) is an intermediate airway allowing ventilation but not complete respiratory control. The LMA consists of an inflatable cuff (the mask) with a connecting tube. It may be used temporarily before tracheal intubation or when tracheal intubation can't be done. It can also be a conduit for later blind insertion of an endotracheal tube. The head and neck must be in neutral position for insertion of the LMA. If the patient has a gag reflex, conscious sedation or topical anesthesia (deep oropharyngeal) is required. The LMA is inserted by sliding along the hard palate, using the finger as a guide, into the pharynx, and the ring is inflated to create a seal about the opening to the larynx, allowing ventilation with mild positive-pressure. The ProSeal® LMA has a modified cuff that extends onto the back of the mask to improve seal. LMA is contraindicated in morbid obesity, obstructions or abnormalities of oropharynx, and non-fasting children, as some aspiration is possible even with the cuff seal inflated.
- A **nasal cannula** can be used to deliver supplemental oxygen to a child, but it is only useful for flow rates ≤6 L/min as higher rates are drying of the nasal passages. Since it is not an airtight system, some ambient air is breathed in as well, so oxygen concentration ranges from about 24–44%. The nasal cannula does not allow for control of respiratory rate, so the child must be able to breathe independently.
- A **non-rebreather mask** can be used to deliver higher concentrations (60–90%) of oxygen to those children who are able to breathe independently. The mask fits over the nose and mouth and is secured by an elastic strap. A 1.5 L reservoir bag is attached and connects to an oxygen source. The bag is inflated to about 1 L at a rate of 8–15 L/min before the mask is applied as the patient breathes from this reservoir. A one-way exhalation valve prevents most exhaled air from being rebreathed.

Radiant warmers

Radiant warmers are devices that provide overhead heat directly to an infant. Radiant heaters provide an area for direct observation and free access to the infant, which is very useful in the initial evaluation and resuscitation (if necessary) of the newborn, or for procedures such as intubation or line placement. Radiant heat devices work best if the room temperature is kept above 25°C. Two problems related to radiant warmers include:

- Promote dehydration if an infant is placed under them for a prolonged amount of time, especially if the infant is premature.
- Risk overheating the infant or causing first-degree burns.

Temperature sensors must be appropriately placed and the infant's temperature monitored frequently to ensure the infant is not being over- or under-heated.

Skin temperature probes

Skin temperature probes are often used to monitor the temperature of the infant in an isolette or radiant warmer. Incorrect placement of the probe can alter the reading, causing the warming device to deliver too much or too little heat. The temperature probe should not be placed over a bony area of the body or over an area where brown adipose tissue is abundant. Brown adipose tissue is abundant around the neck, the mid-scapular region of the back, the mediastinum and organs in the thoracic cavity, kidneys, and adrenal glands. A common probe placement area for an infant who is supine is over the liver. If the probe is not making good skin contact, it will indicate that the infant is cold, and the warmer will deliver increased amounts of heat, possibly causing hyperthermia. If the probe is underneath the infant, it may indicate an artificially warm temperature and decrease heat to the infant, causing hypothermia.

Management of foreign body aspiration

Infants and children, especially those weak or ill, are prone to **aspiration of foreign substances** (food, powder, secretions) or objects (dry nuts, candy, popcorn, toys). Small children, especially, tend to put almost anything into their mouths. Round foods, such as candies, hot dogs, or foods not easily chewed, such as apples, carrots, or hard cookies are especially dangerous. Aspirated foreign bodies are rarely coughed up and must be removed.

Symptoms	Treatment
Initial: Severe coughing, gagging, sternal retraction, wheezing. Objects in the larynx may cause inability to breathe or speak and may lead to respiratory arrest. If the aspirant lodges in the bronchus, cough, dyspnea, and wheezing occur. **Delayed:** Hours, days, or weeks later, an undetected aspirant may cause an infection distal to the aspirated material. Symptoms depend on the area and extent of the infection.	Laryngoscopy or bronchoscopy for removal of object Antibiotic therapy for secondary infection Symptomatic treatment for respiratory distress as indicated

Patient and Family Care: Medical emergencies

Airway

Anaphylaxis syndrome

Anaphylaxis syndrome may present with a few symptoms or a wide range that encompasses cardiopulmonary, dermatological, and gastrointestinal responses. Symptoms may recur after the initial treatment (biphasic anaphylaxis) in about 6% of children, so careful monitoring is essential.

Symptoms	Treatment
Sudden onset of weakness, dizziness, confusion Severe generalized edema and angioedema; lips and tongue may swell Urticaria Increased permeability of vascular system and loss of vascular tone Severe hypotension leading to shock Laryngospasm/bronchospasm with obstruction of airway causing dyspnea and wheezing Nausea, vomiting, and diarrhea Seizures, coma, and death	Establish patent airway and intubate if necessary for ventilation. Provide oxygen at 100% high flow. Monitor VS. Administer epinephrine (Epi-Pen® or 1:1000 solution 0.1 mg/kg to maximum 0.3 mg). Albuterol 2.5 mg (or 0.5%) per nebulizer for bronchospasm Intravenous fluids to provide bolus of fluids for hypotension Diphenhydramine 1.0 mg/kg (to maximum of 50 mg) if shock persists Methylprednisolone 2.0 mg/kg if no response to other drugs

Acute epiglottitis

Acute epiglottitis (supraglottitis) occurs in children primarily from 1–8 years of age although it can occur at any age. It requires immediate medical attention as it can rapidly become obstructive. The onset is usually very sudden and often occurs during the night. The child may awaken suddenly with a fever, but usually does not have a cough. The symptoms include:

- **Tripod position:** Child sits upright, leaning forward with chin out, mouth open, and tongue protruding.
- **Agitation:** The child appears restless, tense, and agitated.
- **Drooling:** Excess secretions combined with pain or dysphagia and mouth open position cause drooling.
- **Voice:** No hoarseness, but voice sounds thick and "froglike."
- **Cyanosis:** Color is usually pale and sallow initially but may progress to frank cyanosis.
- **Throat:** On examination, the epiglottis appears bright red and swollen. NOTE: the child's throat should not be examined with a tongue blade unless intubation and tracheostomy equipment is immediately available as the examination can trigger obstruction.

Tracheal stenosis

Tracheal stenosis is a marked narrowing of the trachea caused by a congenital malformation or trauma, such as from long-term intubation. Congenital tracheal stenosis may not be evident at birth, but may appear later as the child develops a respiratory infection that further impinges on the airway and exhibits signs of respiratory distress, such as cough, wheezing, and biphasic stridor.

Children with tracheal stenosis often hyperextend the neck because this helps to open the airway. Diagnosis is per bronchoscopy although CT or MRI may also be used if severe stenosis precludes bronchoscopy. Treatment for mild stenosis includes a series of tracheal dilations with dilators or rigid bronchoscopy in increasing sizes. Complications of dilation include perforation and airway obstruction (blood, edema). Medications to reduce edema obstruction include epinephrine and corticosteroids. With severe stenosis, tracheostomy, tracheal reconstruction with stents, or tracheal resection may be necessary.

Tracheomalacia

Congenital tracheomalacia is a condition in which the tracheal cartilage is not fully developed at birth so that the trachea is not stable. The degree of respiratory impairment depends on the extent of the abnormality. In most cases, the cartilage develops adequately by 2 years, and surgical repair, which can include tracheostomy, stent placement, and repair of underlying cause, is rarely necessary. Diagnosis is per laryngoscopy.

Symptoms	Treatment
Symptoms may be mild to severe and include: Noisy, audible breathing sounds, especially when position changed Dyspnea, respiratory distress High-pitched or rattling breathing sounds	Treatment includes conservative measures: Providing humidified air Elevating child's head and upper body for feeding to prevent aspiration Feeding slowly Providing chest physiotherapy Controlling infections with antibiotics as indicated

Pneumothorax

Pneumothorax is the most common type of air leak syndrome. In infants, increased air pressure caused by the use of mechanical ventilation is the most common cause, but infants may develop spontaneous pneumothorax. Infants with fragile lung tissue are at high risk.
Infants with lung disease, including hyaline membrane disease (HMD)
Premature infants
Infants with meconium aspiration
Additionally, 5% of children hospitalized for asthma experience pneumothorax as do 10–25% of children >10 years old with cystic fibrosis. Pneumothorax may also occur with thoracic trauma.

Symptoms	Treatment
Increased respiratory distress with tachypnea and chest wall retractions Absence of breath sounds on auscultation Paradoxical chest movement in which the chest contracts during inhalation and expands during exhalation Shift in maximum intensity sounds of heart Bradycardia and cyanosis	Evacuating air with needle aspiration or chest tubes to water seal drainage Correction of underlying cause

Respiratory (Upper and Lower)

Aspiration pneumonia

Aspiration pneumonia may occur as the result of any type of aspiration, including foreign objects. The aspirated material creates an inflammatory response, with the irritated mucous membrane at high risk for bacterial infection secondary to the aspiration. With infants and small children who are weak or suffer from paralysis or congenital anomalies or lack adequate cough reflex, the most common causes of aspiration pneumonia are fluids or foods. Children with respiratory stress or crying during feeding can easily aspirate. Talcum powder used during diaper changes is also implicated. Toddlers and young children may aspirate lighter fluids or other hydrocarbon liquids. Symptoms are similar to other pneumonia, depending upon the site of inflammation: cough, dyspnea, respiratory distress, and cyanosis. Treatment includes:

- Removal of foreign object if indicated (laryngoscopy/bronchoscopy)
- Antibiotic therapy as indicated
- Symptomatic respiratory support
- Preventive methods to avoid aspiration, such as careful feeding and positioning child on the right side after feeding

Pulmonary embolism

Pulmonary embolism, rare in children, can occur with trauma, burns, central lines, catheters, shock, sepsis, immunosuppression, and surgery. Many occurrences are essentially silent. Diagnosis in children is usually with ventilation perfusion scans, CT, pulmonary angiography, or MRI.

Symptoms	Treatment
Dyspnea with tachypnea (less common than with adults). Tachycardia. Anxiety. Pleuritic pain. Fever. Rales. Cough (sometimes with hemoptysis). Hemodynamic instability. Friction rub.	Oxygen. Intravenous infusions. Dobutamine (Dobutrex®) or dopamine (Intropin®) for hypotension. Cardiac monitoring for dysrhythmias. Medications as indicated: digitalis glycosides, diuretics, and antiarrhythmics. Intubation and mechanical ventilation if needed. Analgesia (such as morphine sulfate) or sedation for anxiety. Anticoagulants to prevent recurrence (although it will not dissolve clots already present), including heparin and warfarin (Coumadin®). Placement of percutaneous venous filter (Greenfield) in the inferior vena cava to prevent further emboli from entering the lungs. Thrombolytic therapy, recombinant tissue-type plasminogen activator (t-PA) or streptokinase, for those severely compromised, but these treatments have limited success and pose the danger of bleeding.

Bronchiolitis (RSV)

Bronchiolitis is inflammation of the bronchiolar level and is usually caused by the **respiratory syncytial virus** (RSV) although adenoviruses, parainfluenza, and *M. pneumoniae* have also been implicated. It is most common in very small children between the ages of 2 months and 2 years and rarely occurs after that age. Most children who require hospitalization are infants under 6 months of age. The infection is usually seasonal and mild although it can result in severe respiratory complications, so children should be observed carefully.

Symptoms	Treatment
Dyspnea, tachypnea, and wheezing Paroxysmal cough that is non-productive Note: The infection is usually self-limiting and runs its course in 8–15 days but is highly contagious.	**Note:** Treatment is primarily symptomatic: Antipyretics, such as acetaminophen Oxygen therapy with intubation and mechanical ventilation may be required in the presence of severe disease and respiratory compromise. Ribavirin aerosol is used for severe disease.

Reactive airway disease

Reactive airway disease is a classification of symptoms rather than a specific diagnosis. Reactive airway disease is characterized by wheezing, coughing, and dyspnea. Often, the symptoms are caused by asthma, but sometimes there are other causes, so asthma and reactive airway disease are not interchangeable terms. Less than a third of young children (<3 years old) who wheeze go on to develop asthma. Reactive airway disease is highest among African Americans and Hispanics. Causes of reactive airway disease can include:

Infection: Narrows airways and weak diaphragm result in compromise.

Environmental allergens: Result in an antibody response that causes inflammation of the airways with resultant edema and bronchospasm.

Rhinoviruses: Cause exacerbation of symptoms in children with asthma.

Environmental exposure to smoke: Increases risk of developing reactive airway disease, especially if the mother smokes during pregnancy and first year.

When a child is classified as having reactive airway disease, the primary goal of diagnostic testing is to identify the underlying cause and the specific disease process causing the symptoms.

Indications of acute respiratory infections

Pediatric manifestations of acute respiratory infections	
Fever	Usually absent in neonates but is highest in those from 6 months to 3 years of age, and may reach 103°F –105°F. Sudden temperature rises to 104° may result in seizures in children <3–4 years of age. Fever may result in some children being listless and others hyperactive.
Lymph Nodes	May be tender and enlarged
Meningeal Irritation	Occurs in some children without meningitis in the presence of an abrupt increase in fever and may manifest with headaches, nuchal rigidity, and pain, as well as positive Kernig and Brudzinski signs: Positive Kernig sign: Flex each hip and then try to straighten the knee while the hip is flexed. Spasm of the hamstrings makes this painful and difficult. Positive Brudzinski sign: With child lying supine, flex the neck by pulling head toward chest. The neck stiffness causes the hips and knees to pull up into a flexed position.
Nasal	May include swelling of nasal passages, causing obstruction that can interfere with feeding in small infants. Exudate may be thin and watery or thick and purulent, depending upon the type of infection. Irritation about the nares and upper lip related to exudate is common in infants and small children.
Sore throat	Usually a complaint of older children. Small infants and children may have an inflamed throat but appear to suffer less discomfort.
Cough	Common symptom that may occur only during the acute phase of the respiratory infection or may persist for months after initial infection.
Respiratory sounds	May include wheezing and hoarseness in addition to cough. On auscultation, abnormal sounds may occur, such as hyperresonance, fine to coarse rales, wheezing, or absence of breath sounds in areas of the lungs.

Manifestations of acute respiratory infections

Pediatric manifestations of acute respiratory infections: Gastrointestinal symptoms	
Poor appetite/ feeding	Often the initial symptom and may persist throughout the febrile and convalescent period. This is a common symptom of acute infection in children.
Nausea & vomiting	May occur before other symptoms by several hours and usually subsides fairly quickly although it may persist with some children. It is most common in small children.
Diarrhea	Common with respiratory infections, especially those of viral origin. In most children, diarrhea is mild and short lasting, but in others it may be severe and increase dehydration.
Abdominal pain	May be related to muscle spasms from vomiting or lymphadenitis of mesentery, especially if the child is very tense. The type of pain may be similar to or indistinguishable from pain associated with appendicitis.

Asthma

Asthma is a chronic reversible or partially reversible inflammation of the airway (especially the lower airways) that results in obstruction associated with genetic predisposition, environmental exposures, viral illnesses, and allergens. Children usually experience the first asthma attack between ages 3 and 8. In some cases, children may complain of a prodromal itch in the neck or upper part of the back prior to an episode. Children's asthma is characterized by increased airway reactivity with obstruction related to inflammation and edema of mucous membranes, accumulation of secretions, and spasms of the smooth muscles of the bronchi and bronchioles. This bronchial constriction increases airway resistance that results in forced expiration through the constricted lumens. Symptoms may include dyspnea, inspiratory and expiratory high-pitched wheezing, cough, prolonged expiration, anxiety, sweating, and cyanosis. Wheezing and crackles may be heard throughout lung fields. Older children often sit upright with shoulders hunched over. Initial cough is usually hacking and nonproductive but then becomes productive of frothy gelatinous sputum. The 3 primary symptoms of asthma are cough, wheezing, and dyspnea.

Assessment criteria for severity of asthma attacks

Assessment criteria for severity of asthma attacks	
Mild	Peak expiratory flow rate (PEFR) 70–90% of normal. Respiratory rate ≤30% above average. Remains alert and no cyanosis or pallor. Dyspnea: Mild or absent with no or mild intercostal retractions. Pulsus paradoxus <10 mm Hg. Oxygen saturation >95% and PCO2 <35. End expiratory wheeze only on auscultation.
Moderate	PEFR 50–70% of normal. Respiratory rate 30–50% above average. Remains alert but pale. Moderate dyspnea but can speak in phrases. Moderate intercostal retractions with tracheosternal retractions and use of accessory muscles. Pulsus paradoxus 10–20 mm Hg. Oxygen saturation 90–95% and PCO2 <40. Inspiratory and expiratory wheeze on auscultation.
Severe	PEFR <50% of normal. Respiratory rate >50% above average. Less alert and may be cyanotic. Severe dyspnea with difficulty speaking and severe retractions with nasal flaring and hyperinflation of chest. Pulsus paradoxus 20–40 mm Hg. Oxygen saturation <90% and PCO2 <40. Breath sounds increasingly inaudible.

Exercise-induced asthma

Exercise-induced asthma (bronchospasm) is especially a risk for those with pre-existing asthma or allergies, especially with high pollen counts, high levels of smog, and cold dry weather. Children usually begin to cough, wheeze, and complain of shortness of breath and chest tightness after about 5 minutes of exercise. The symptoms may increase 5 to 10 minutes after exercise ceases, but symptoms usually recede by 30 minutes. Children should be cautioned to regularly take all prescribed preventive medications and warm up for 5 to 10 minutes before doing strenuous exercise. Additionally, they should breathe through their noses to warm the air and learn to monitor their own breathing. Immediate care includes stopping activity, positioning person in upright position, and having the athlete use his/her inhaled bronchodilator. If symptoms are severe and do not begin to subside after ceasing activity and using bronchodilator, the child may require emergent treatment.

Status asthmaticus

Status asthmaticus is a severe acute attack of asthma that does not respond to conventional therapy, such as inhaled bronchodilators, and progresses to respiratory failure. The child with status asthmaticus will often present in acute distress, nonresponsive to inhaled bronchodilators. Airway obstruction, sternal and intercostal retractions

Tachypnea and dyspnea, increasing cyanosis
Forced prolonged expirations
Cardiac decompensation with increased left ventricular afterload and increased pulmonary edema resulting from alveolar-capillary permeability. Hypoxia may trigger an increase in pulmonary vascular resistance with increased right ventricular afterload.
Pulsus paradoxus (decreased pulse on inspiration and increased on expiration) with extra beats on inspiration detected through auscultation but not detected radially. Blood pressure normally decreases slightly during inspiration, but this response is exaggerated. Pulsus paradoxus indicates increasing severity of asthma.
Hypoxemia (with impending respiratory failure)
Hypocapnia followed by hypercapnia (with impending respiratory failure)
Metabolic acidosis

Mechanical ventilation

Mechanical ventilation (MV) for status asthmaticus should be avoided if possible because of the danger of increased bronchospasm as well as barotrauma and decreased circulation. Aggressive medical management with β-adrenergic agonists, corticosteroids, and anticholinergics should be tried prior to ventilation. However, there are some absolute indications for the use of intubation and ventilation and a number of other indications that are evaluated on an individual basis.

Absolute indications for MV	Relative indications for MV
Cardiac and/or pulmonary arrest. Markedly depressed mental status (obtundation). Severe hypoxia and/or apnea. Bradycardia.	Exhaustion/ muscle fatigue from exertion of trying to breathe. Sharply diminished breath sounds and no audible wheezing. Pulse Pulsus paradoxus >20–40 mm Hg. If pulsus paradoxus is absent, this is an indication of imminent respiratory arrest. PaO_2 <70 mm Hg on 100% oxygen. Deteriorating mental status. Dysphonia. Central cyanosis. Increased hypercapnia. Metabolic/respiratory acidosis: pH <7.20

Pneumonia: Overview

Pneumonia is inflammation of the lung parenchyma, filling the alveoli with exudate. It is common throughout childhood and adulthood but more frequent in infants and young children. Pneumonia may be a primary disease or may occur secondary to another infection or disease, such as lung cancer. Pneumonia may be caused by bacteria, viruses, parasites, or fungi. It may also be caused by chemical damage. Pneumonia is characterized by location.

- **Lobar** involves one or more lobes of the lungs. If lobes in both lungs are affected, it is referred to as "bilateral" or "double" pneumonia.
- **Bronchial/lobular** involves the terminal bronchioles and exudate can involve the adjacent lobules. Usually the pneumonia occurs in scattered patches throughout the lungs.
- **Interstitial** involves primarily the interstitium and alveoli where white blood cells and plasma fill the alveoli, generating inflammation and creating fibrotic tissue as the alveoli are destroyed.

Community-acquired pneumonia

Streptococcus pneumoniae (a Gram-positive coccus) is part of the normal flora of the upper respiratory tract and is the most frequent cause of bacterial pneumonia, often secondary to an upper respiratory tract infection. The overall incidence has dropped since the heptavalent pneumococcal conjugate vaccine (PCV-7) was introduced in 2000, with the most significant effect on those under 2 years of age (78% drop in cases); however, a vaccinated infant that is febrile with toxic symptoms and a leukocyte count of ≥15,000 cells/mL is at risk for pneumonia. The bacteria induce an acute inflammatory response causing the alveoli and interstitium to fill with protein-rich fluid. The infection spreads quickly, often to multiple lobes, causing consolidation; pleural effusions, super infections, bacteremia (15–25%) and pericarditis may occur. Symptoms include an abrupt onset with high fever (≥105°), chills, diaphoresis, cyanosis, chest pain, tachypnea, tachycardia, altered consciousness, and cough productive of rusty or green-tinged mucus. Treatment may include:

- Antipyretics, Analgesics
- Respiratory support
- Antibiotics: penicillins or others

Haemophilus influenzae frequently colonizes the upper respiratory tracts in children <5 and can lead to pneumonia. However, in 1990, the conjugated polysaccharide *H. influenzae* type B vaccine was introduced, and this has greatly decreased the incidence of pneumonia in small children. Non-type B and nontypeable cases of *H. influenzae* pneumonia do occur. This pneumonia is similar in symptoms to other bacterial forms, but the onset is often slow and insidious, appearing 2–6 weeks after an upper respiratory tract infection. Symptoms include fever, chills, and productive cough. The disease may occur as lobar or bronchial pneumonia or with areas of consolidation where the alveoli have collapsed and the tissue hardened. Complications may include bacteremia, lung abscesses, pleural effusions, epiglottitis, and pericarditis. Treatment is symptomatic and may include:

- Antipyretics, such as acetaminophen or ibuprofen
- Analgesics
- Respiratory support
- Antibiotics: ampicillin, 3rd generation cephalosporin, macrolides

Mycoplasma pneumoniae are pleomorphic (variously shaped) microorganisms that interfere with the function of the cilia and produce hydrogen peroxide, which disrupts cell functions. The organisms also activate an inflammatory response. Only about 3% of those infected develop pneumonia, affecting primarily children and young adults between the ages of 4 and 20. *Mycoplasma pneumoniae* infection occurs seasonally in the fall in a regular 4 to 8 year cycle of epidemics. The onset is usually gradual, and children tend to be less obviously ill than with other types of pneumonia. Symptoms may include a paroxysmal cough, low-grade fever, myalgia, diarrhea, erythematous rash, and pharyngitis. The pneumonia presents as interstitial infiltrates on x-ray. While complications, such as myocarditis, endocarditis, aseptic meningitis, and encephalitis may occur, most infections clear without sequelae. Treatment includes:
Antibiotic therapy: erythromycin, tetracycline, macrolide, or fluoroquinolone
Symptomatic support: antidiarrheals, antipyretics, and analgesics

Viral pneumonia

Viral pneumonia is more common in adults than children although the respiratory syncytial virus (RSV), which causes upper respiratory infections and bronchiolitis can progress to pneumonia and is most commonly found in children ≤5. A number of other viruses, such as adenoviruses, parainfluenza, cytomegalovirus, and coronavirus may be implicated. The viruses invade the cells that line the airways and alveoli, causing death of the cells. Symptoms related to viral pneumonia are similar to those of bacterial pneumonia although the onset is often slow with pneumonia preceded by a respiratory infection that progressively worsens, with increasing cough, fever, dyspnea, cyanosis, and respiratory distress. There are few effective treatments for viral pneumonia, and one danger is that a viral pneumonia increases susceptibility to bacterial infection of the lungs. Treatment may include:

- Rest and adequate fluids and nutrition
- Antipyretics, such as acetaminophen or ibuprofen
- Oxygen therapy with intubation and mechanical ventilation may be required in the presence of severe disease and respiratory compromise.
- Ribavirin aerosol is used for severe RSV disease and pneumonia.

Cardiac tamponade

Cardiac tamponade occurs with pericardial effusion in which fluid accumulates in the pericardial sac, causing pressure against the heart. It may be a complication of trauma, pericarditis, cardiac surgery, or heart failure. Fluid normally circulates in the pericardial area to reduce friction, and a sudden increase in this volume can compress the heart causing a number of cardiac responses:

- Increased end-diastolic pressure in both ventricles
- Decrease in venous return
- Decrease in ventricular filling

Symptoms may include a feeling of pressure or pain in the chest as well as dyspnea, and pulsus paradoxus >10 mm Hg (systolic blood pressure heard during exhalation but not during inhalation). Beck's triad (increased central venous pressure with distended neck veins, muffled heart sounds, and hypotension) is commonly found. Treatment includes pericardiocentesis with large bore needle or surgical repair to control bleeding and relieve cardiac compression.

Bronchopulmonary dysplasia

Bronchopulmonary dysplasia (BPD) is a chronic lung disease characterized by alveolar damage resulting from abnormal development with inflammation and development of scar tissue. Risk factors include:
Prematurity of >10 weeks prior to due date
Birthweight <2.5 lbs./1000 grams
Hyaline membrane disease or respiratory distress syndrome (RDS) at birth
Long-term ventilatory support/oxygen
Most of the infants have immature lungs with inadequate surfactant to allow the lungs to expand properly, so they cannot breathe without assistance. Symptoms include severe respiratory distress and cyanosis. Usually infants improve within 2–4 weeks with treatment, but some progress from RDS to BPD. Their lungs often have fewer but enlarged alveoli with inadequate blood supply. BPD is usually diagnosed if respiratory symptoms do not improve after 28 days.

Bronchopulmonary dysplasia (BPD)	
Treatment	**Complications**
Supportive treatment provides oxygenation, protects vital organs, and allows the lungs to mature: Surfactant. Nasal continuous positive airway pressure (NCPAP). Mechanical ventilation or high-frequency jet ventilation (HFJV). Supplemental oxygen. Bronchodilators (albuterol) to open airways. Furosemide (Lasix®) to reduce pulmonary edema. Antibiotics as indicated. Gastric /enteral feedings or total parenteral nutrition (TPN).	Most infants are hospitalized for about 4 months but may need treatment for months or years at home. Most will eventually develop nearly normal lung function as new lung tissue grows and takes over the function of the scarred tissue. Some long-term complications may occur: Increased risk of bacterial and viral infections, such as RSV and pneumonia. Chronic or recurrent pulmonary edema. Pulmonary hypertension. Side effects related to long-term use of diuretics, such as hearing deficits, renal calculi, and electrolyte imbalances. Slow growth patterns.

Cardiovascular

Tension pneumothorax

Pneumothorax is a leak between the lung tissue and the chest wall so extraneous air is in the pleural space. **Tension pneumothorax** is similar to traumatic open pneumothorax; however, the air can enter the pleural sac but can't be expelled. Air enters the sac from lacerations in a lung or opening into the chest wall. Because the air is trapped and cannot be expelled, with each breath the positive pressure in the pleural sac increases, resulting in collapse of the lung and a pronounced mediastinal shift to the unaffected side with severe compromise of cardiac and respiratory function. The increasing pressure decreases venous return, resulting in decreased cardiac output and reduced peripheral circulation. Open wounds must be sealed, and chest tubes inserted to drain air and fluid. In some cases, needle decompression is done prior to chest tube insertion. Supplemental oxygen (high concentration) should be administered and pulse oximetry monitored.

Cardiogenic shock

Cardiogenic shock in children usually relates to congenital heart disease (usually with systemic to pulmonary shunting), myocarditis, and dysrhythmias, such as AV block and paroxysmal atrial tachycardia. It may also indicate end-stage sepsis, muscular dystrophy, and hypoglycemia. These disorders interfere with the pumping mechanism of the heart, decreasing oxygen perfusion. Cardiogenic shock has 3 characteristics: increased preload, increased afterload, and decreased contractibility. These result in decreased cardiac output and increased systemic vascular resistance (SVR) to compensate and protect vital organs, causing increased afterload in the left ventricle with increased need for oxygen. As the cardiac output continues to decrease, tissue perfusion decreases, coronary artery perfusion decreases, fluid backs up and the left ventricle fails to adequately pump the blood, resulting in pulmonary edema and right ventricular failure. Treatment includes:

- Ventilatory support with oxygen (usually 100%), intubation as needed
- Treatment of underlying condition (antibiotics, glucose)
- Antiarrhythmics
- Diuretics (furosemide)
- Fluid management (intravenous)
- Inotropic agents (often epinephrine 1:1000, 0.1 mg/k to maximum 0.5 mg)

Sinus bradycardia

There are 3 primary types of **sinus node dysrhythmias**: sinus bradycardia, sinus tachycardia, and sinus arrhythmia**. Sinus bradycardia (SB)** is caused by a decreased rate of impulse from sinus node. The pulse and ECG usually appear normal except for a slower rate.

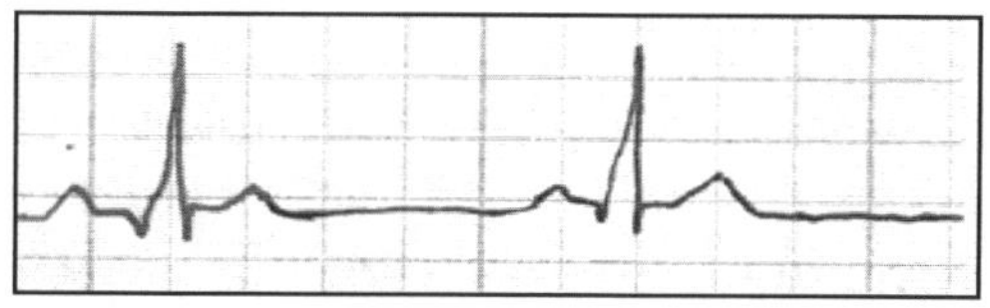

SB is characterized by a regular pulse <50 to 60 with P waves in front of QRS, which are usually normal in shape and duration. PR interval is 0.12 to 0.20 seconds, QRS interval 0.04 to 0.11 seconds, and P:QRS ratio of 1:1. SB may be caused by a number of factors:

- Conditions that lower the body's metabolic needs, such as hypothermia or sleep
- Hypotension and decrease in oxygenation
- Medications such as calcium channel blockers and β-blockers

- Vagal stimulation that may result from vomiting, suctioning, or defecating
- Increased intracranial pressure
- Myocardial infarction

Treatment involves eliminating cause if possible, such as changing medications. Atropine may be given IV to block vagal stimulation.

Sinus tachycardia

Sinus tachycardia (ST) occurs when the sinus node impulse increases in frequency. ST is characterized by a regular pulse >100 with P waves before QRS but sometimes part of preceding T wave. QRS is usually of normal shape and duration (0.04 to 0.11 seconds) but may have consistent irregularity. PR interval is 0.12–0.20 seconds and P:QRS ratio of 1:1.

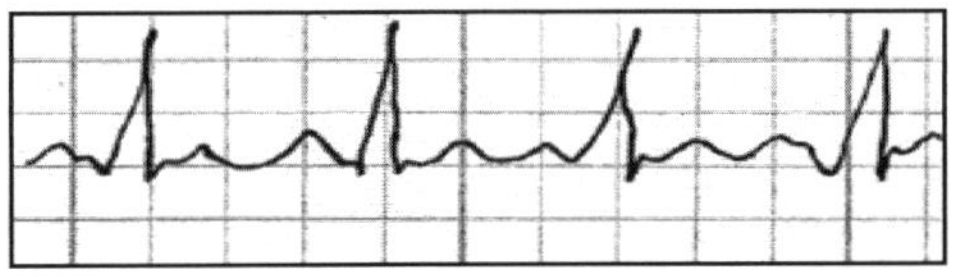

The rapid pulse decreases diastolic filling time and causes reduced cardiac output with resultant hypotension. Acute pulmonary edema may result from the decreased ventricular filling if untreated. ST may be caused by a number of factors:

- Acute blood loss, shock, hypovolemia, anemia
- Sinus arrhythmia, hypovolemic heart failure
- Hypermetabolic conditions, fever, infection
- Exertion/exercise, anxiety
- Medications, such as sympathomimetic drugs

Treatment includes eliminating precipitating factors and administering calcium channel blockers and β-blockers to reduce heart rate.

Supraventricular tachycardia

Supraventricular tachycardia (SVT) (>100 BPM) may have a sudden onset and result in congestive heart failure. Rate may increase to 200 to 300 BPM. SVT originates in the atria rather than the ventricles but is controlled by the tissue in the area of the AV node rather than the SA node. Rhythm is usually rapid but regular. The P wave is present but may not be clearly defined as it may be obscured by the preceding T wave, and the QRS complex appears normal. The PR interval is 0.12 to 0.20 seconds and QRS interval 0.04 to 0.11 seconds with P:QRS ratio of 1:1. SVT may be episodic with periods of normal heart rate and rhythm between episodes of SVT, so it is often referred to as paroxysmal SVT (PSVT).

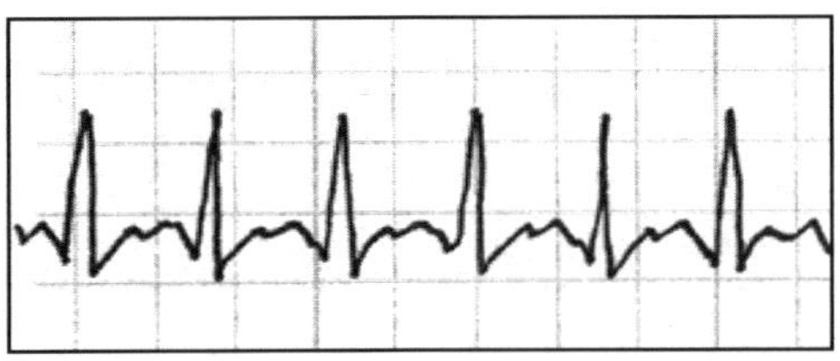

Sinus arrhythmia

Sinus arrhythmia (SA) results from irregular impulses from the sinus node, often paradoxical (increasing with inspiration and decreasing with expiration) because of stimulation of the vagal nerve during inspiration and rarely causes a negative hemodynamic effect. These cyclic changes in the pulse during respiration are quite common in both children and young adults and often lessen with

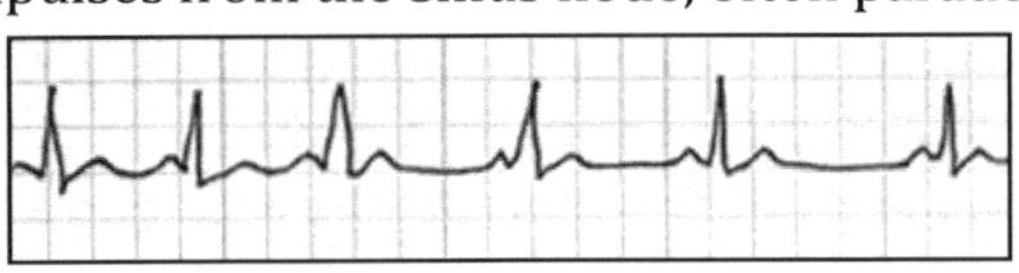

age but may persist in some adults. Sinus arrhythmia can, in some cases, relate to heart or valvular disease and may be increased with vagal stimulation for suctioning, vomiting, or defecating. Characteristics of SA include a regular pulse 50–100, P waves in front of QRS with duration (0.4 to 0.11 seconds) and shape of QRS usually normal, PR interval of 0.12 to 0.20 seconds, and P:QRS ratio of 1:1. Treatment is usually not necessary unless it is associated with bradycardia.

Premature atrial contractions

There are 3 primary types of **atrial dysrhythmias**, including premature atrial contractions, atrial flutter, and atrial fibrillation. **Premature atrial contraction (PAC)** is essentially an extra beat precipitated by an electrical impulse to the atrium before the sinus node impulse. The extra beat may be caused by alcohol, caffeine, nicotine, hypervolemia, hypokalemia, hypermetabolic conditions, atrial ischemia or infarction. Characteristics include an irregular pulse because of extra P waves, shape and duration of QRS is usually normal (0.04 to 0.11 seconds) but may be abnormal, PR interval remains between 0.12 to 0.20, and P:QRS ratio is 1:1. Rhythm is irregular with varying P-P and R-R intervals. PACs can occur in an essentially healthy heart and are not usually cause for concern unless they are frequent (>6/hr) and cause severe palpitations. In that case, atrial fibrillation should be suspected.

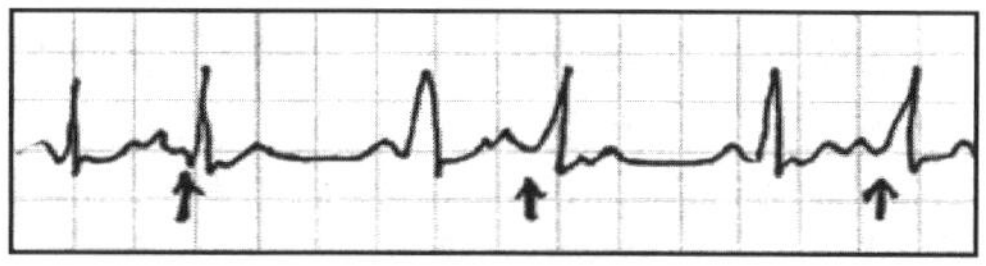

Atrial flutter

Atrial flutter (AF) occurs when the atrial rate is faster, usually 250–400 beats per minute, than the AV node conduction rate so not all of the beats are conducted into the ventricles, effectively blocked at the AV node, preventing ventricular fibrillation although some extra ventricular impulses may go though. AF is caused by the same conditions that cause atrial fibrillation: coronary artery disease, valvular disease, pulmonary disease, heavy alcohol ingestion, and cardiac surgery. AF is characterized by atrial rates of 250–400 with ventricular rates of 75–150, and ventricular rate usually regular. P waves are saw-toothed (referred to as F waves), QRS shape and duration (0.4 to 0.11 seconds) are usually normal, PR interval may be hard to calculate because of F waves, and the P:QRS ratio is 2-4:1. Symptoms include chest pain, dyspnea, and hypotension.

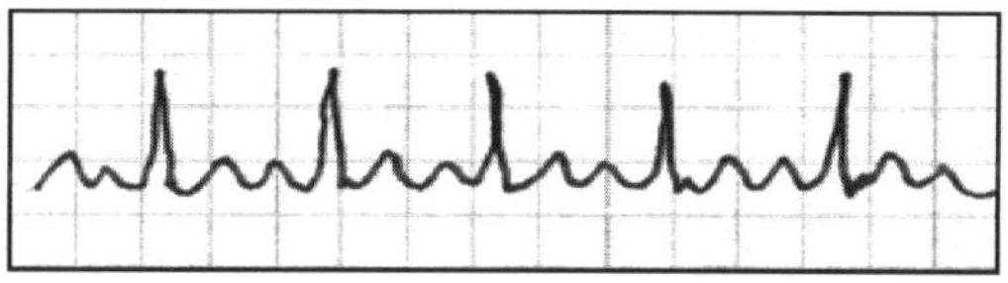

Treatment includes:
Cardioversion if condition is unstable
Medications to slow ventricular rate and conduction through AV node: Cardizem®, Calan®
Medications to convert to sinus rhythm: Corvert®, Cardioquin®, Norpace®, Cordarone®

Atrial fibrillation

Atrial fibrillation (a-fib) is rapid, disorganized atrial beats that are ineffective in emptying the atria, so that blood pools and can lead to thrombus formation and emboli. The ventricular rate increases with a decreased stroke volume, and cardiac output decreases with increased myocardial ischemia, resulting in palpitations and

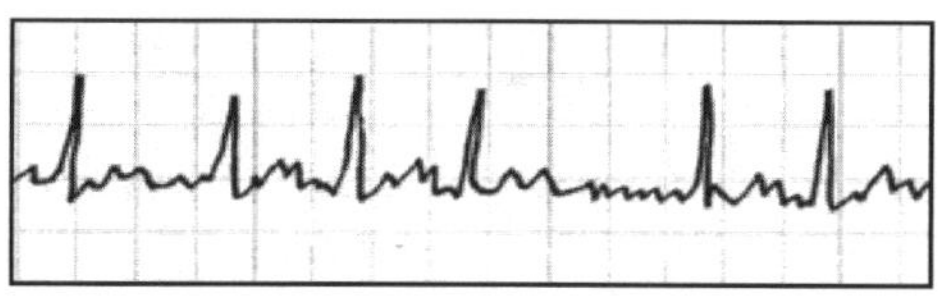

fatigue. A-fib is caused by coronary artery disease, valvular disease, pulmonary disease, heavy alcohol ingestion, and cardiac surgery. A-fib is characterized by very irregular pulse with atrial rate of 300–600 and ventricular rate of 120–200, shape and duration (0.4 to 0.11 seconds) of QRS is usually normal. Fibrillatory (F) waves are seen instead of P waves. The PR interval cannot be measured and the P:QRS ratio is highly variable. Score as a-fib during sleep with irregularly irregular ventricular rhythm and varying rapid oscillations replacing P waves. Medications may include:

- For acute: ibutilide, procainamide, digoxin
- To maintain rhythm: quinidine, amiodarone
- To control ventricular rate: β-blockers, calcium channel blockers, and verapamil
- Anticoagulant therapy

Premature junctional contractions

The area around the AV node is the junction, and dysrhythmias that arise from that are called junctional dysrhythmias. **Premature junctional contractions** (PJCs) occur when a premature impulse starts at the AV node before the next normal sinus impulse reaches the AV node. PJCs are similar to premature atrial contractions (PACs) and generally require no treatment although they may be an indication of digoxin toxicity. The ECG may appear basically normal with an early QRS complex that is normal in shape and duration (0.4 to 0.11 seconds). The P wave may be absent, precede, be part of, or follow the QRS with a PR interval of N0.12 seconds. The P:QRS ratio may vary from <1:1 to 1:1 (with inverted P wave). Rhythm is usually regular at a heart rate of 40 to 60. Significant symptoms related to premature junctional contractions are rare.

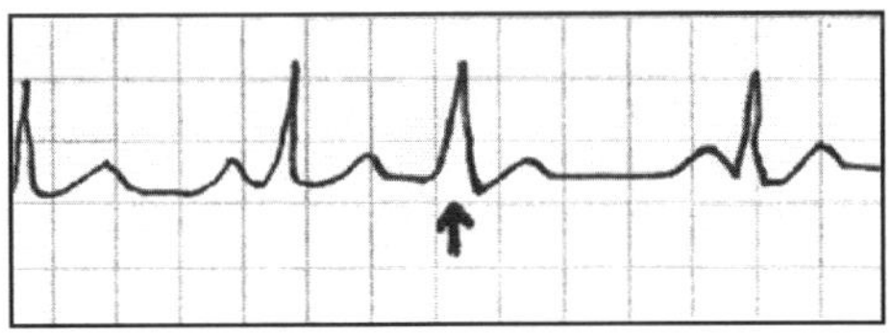

Junctional rhythms

Junctional rhythms occur when the AV node becomes the pacemaker of the heart because the sinus node is depressed from increased vagal tone or a block at the AV node prevents sinus node impulses from being transmitted. While the sinus node normally sends impulses 60–100 beats per minute, the AV node junction usually sends impulses at 40–60 beats per minute. The QRS complex is of usual shape and duration (0.4 to 0.11 seconds). The P wave may be inverted and may be absent, hidden or after the QRS. If the P wave precedes the QRS, the PR interval is <0.12 seconds. The P:QRS ratio is <1:1 or 1:1. The **junctional escape rhythm** is a protective mechanism preventing asystole with failure of the sinus node.

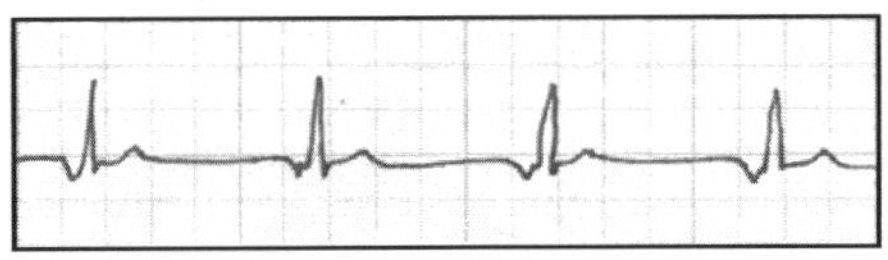

An **accelerated junctional rhythm** is similar, but the heart rate is 60 to 100. **Junctional tachycardia** occurs with heart rate of >100.

AV nodal reentry tachycardia

AV nodal reentry tachycardia occurs when an impulse conducts to area of the AV node, and the impulse is sent in a rapidly repeating cycle back to the same area and to the ventricles, resulting in a fast ventricular rate. The onset and cessation are usually rapid. AV nodal reentry tachycardia (also known as paroxysmal atrial tachycardia or supraventricular tachycardia if no P waves) is characterized by atrial rate of 150–250 with ventricular rate of 75–250, P wave that is difficult to

see or absent, QRS complex that is usually normal and a PR interval of <0.12 if a P wave is present. The P:QRS ratio is 1–2:1. Precipitating factors include nicotine, caffeine, hypoxemia, and anxiety and underlying coronary artery disease and cardiomyopathy. Cardiac output may be decreased with a rapid heart rate, causing dyspnea, chest pain, and hypotension. Treatment may include:
Vagal maneuvers (carotid sinus massage, gag reflex, holding breath)
Medications (adenosine, verapamil, or diltiazem)
Cardioversion if other methods unsuccessful

Premature ventricular contractions

Premature ventricular contractions (PVCs) are those in which the impulse begins in the ventricles and conducts through them prior to the next sinus impulse. The ectopic QRS complexes may vary in shape, depending upon whether there is one site (unifocal) or more (multifocal) that is stimulating the ectopic beats. PVCs usually cause no morbidity unless there is underlying cardiac disease or an acute MI. PVCs are characterized by an irregular heartbeat, QRS that is ≥0.12 seconds and oddly shaped, P wave that may be absent or may precede or follow the QRS, a PR interval of <0.12 seconds if P wave is present, and a P:QRS ratio of 0–1:1. Short-term therapy may include lidocaine, but PVCs are often not treated in otherwise healthy people. PVCs may be precipitated by caffeine, nicotine, or alcohol. Because PVCs may occur with any supraventricular dysrhythmia, the underlying rhythm (such as atrial fibrillation) must be noted as well as the PVCs.

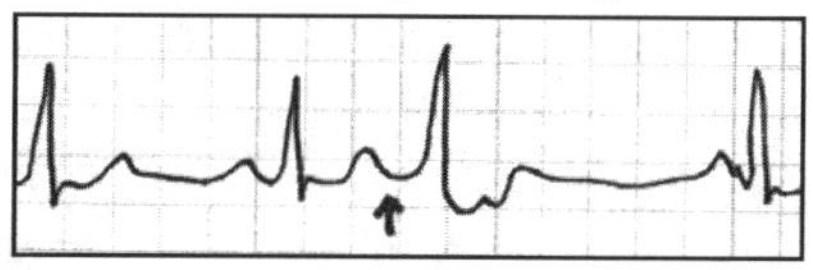

Ventricular tachycardia

Ventricular tachycardia (VT) is ≥3 PVCs in a row with a ventricular rate of 100–200 beats per minute. Ventricular tachycardia may be triggered by the same things as PVCs and is often related to underlying coronary artery disease, but the rapid rate of contractions make VT dangerous as the ineffective beats may render the person unconscious with no palpable pulse. A detectable rate is usually regular and the QRS complex is ≥0.12 seconds and is usually abnormally shaped. The P wave may be undetectable with an irregular PR interval if P wave is present. The P:QRS ratio is often difficult to ascertain because of absence of P waves.

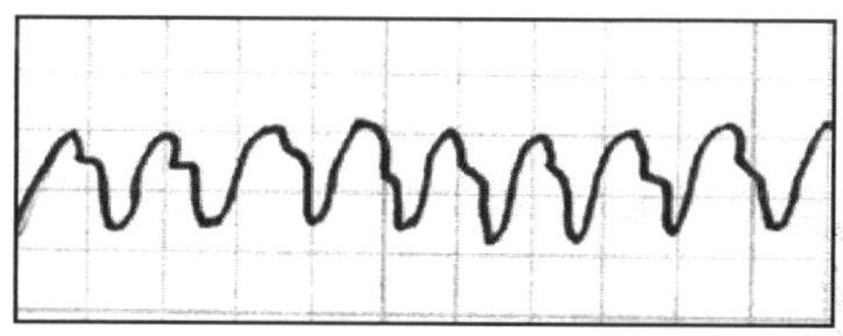

Narrow complex and wide complex tachycardias

Tachycardias are classified as narrow complex or wide complex. Wide and narrow refer to the configuration of the QRS complex :

Wide complex tachycardia: About 80% of cases of WCT are caused by ventricular tachycardia. WCT originates at some point below the AV node and may be associated with palpitations, dyspnea, anxiety, and cardiac arrest. Patients may exhibit diaphoresis. Wide complex tachycardia is diagnosed with ≥3 consecutive beats at a heart rate >100 BPM and QRS duration ≥0.12 seconds.

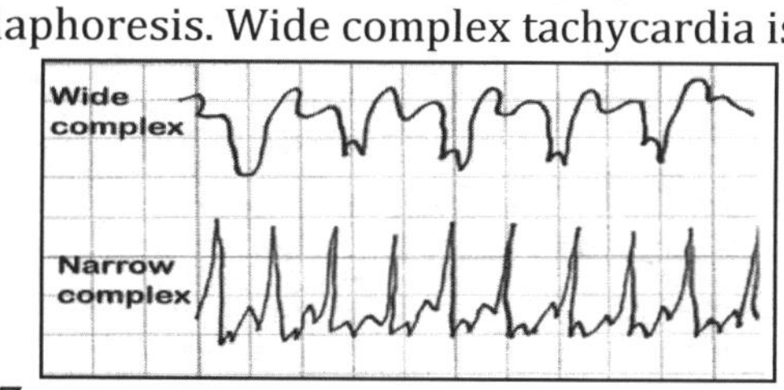

Narrow complex tachycardia: NCT is associated with palpitations, dyspnea, and peripheral edema. NCT is generally supraventricular in origin. Narrow complex tachycardia is diagnosed with ≥3 consecutive beats at heart rate of >100 BPM and QRS duration of <0.12 seconds.

Ventricular fibrillation

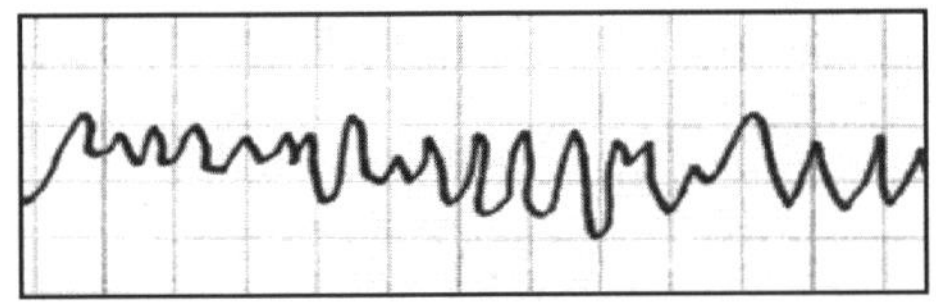

Ventricular fibrillation (VF) is a rapid, very irregular ventricular rate >300 beats per minute with no atrial activity observable on the ECG, caused by disorganized electrical activity in the ventricles. The QRS complex is not recognizable as ECG shows irregular undulations. The causes are the same as for ventricular tachycardia (VT) (alcohol, caffeine, nicotine, underlying coronary disease), and it may result if VT is not treated. It may also result from an electrical shock or congenital disorder, such as Brugada syndrome. VF is accompanied by lack of palpable pulse, audible pulse, and respirations and is immediately life threatening without defibrillation. After emergency defibrillation, the cause should be identified and limited. Mortality is high if VF occurs as part of a myocardial infarction.

Idioventricular rhythm

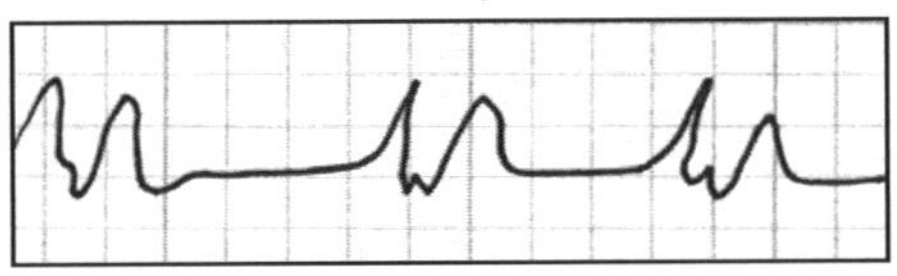

Ventricular escape rhythm (idioventricular) occurs when the Purkinje fibers below the AV node create an impulse. This may occur if the sinus node fails to fire or if there is blockage at the AV node so that the impulse does not go through. Idioventricular rhythm is characterized by a regular ventricular rate of 20–40. Rates >40 are called accelerated idioventricular rhythm. The P wave is missing and the QRS complex has a very bizarre and abnormal shape with duration of ≥0.12 seconds. The low ventricular rate may cause a decrease in cardiac output, often making the patient lose consciousness. In other patients, the idioventricular rhythm may not be associated with reduced cardiac output.

Ventricular asystole

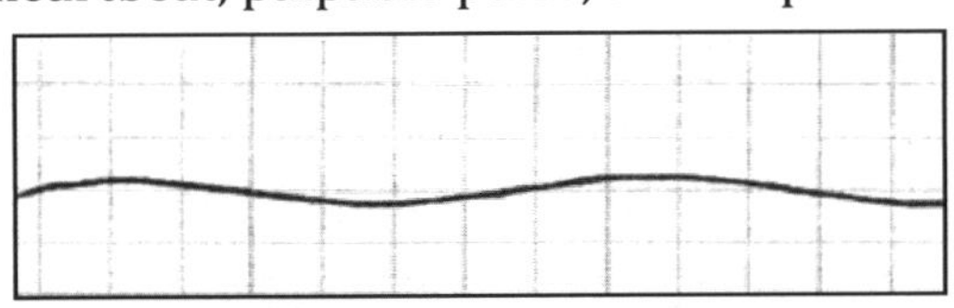

Ventricular asystole is the absence of audible heartbeat, palpable pulse, and respirations, a condition often referred to as "flatlining" or "cardiac arrest." While the ECG may show some P waves initially, the QRS complex is absent although there may be an occasional QRS "escape beat." Cardiopulmonary resuscitation is required with intubation for ventilation and establishment of an intravenous line for fluids. Without immediate treatment, the patient will suffer from severe hypoxia and brain death within minutes. Identifying the cause is critical for the patient's survival and could include hypoxia, acidosis, electrolyte imbalance, hypothermia, or drug overdose. Even with immediate treatment, the prognosis is poor and ventricular asystole is often a sign of impending death.

Sinus pause

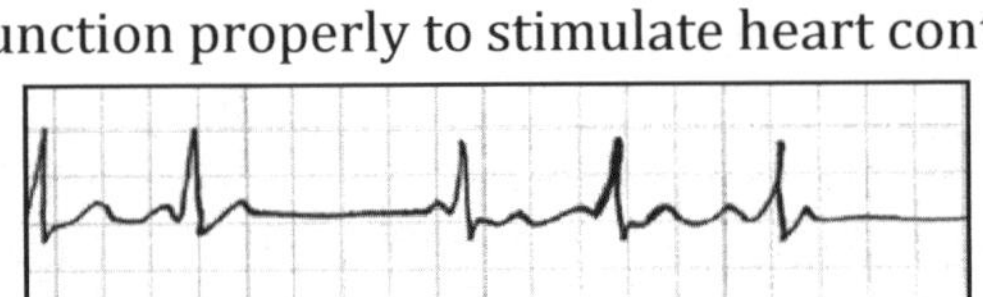

Sinus pause occurs when the sinus node fails to function properly to stimulate heart contractions and the P wave, so there is a pause on the ECG recording that may persist for a few seconds to minutes, depending on the severity of the dysfunction. A prolonged pause may be difficult to differentiate from cardiac arrest, so the technologist should alert medical personnel if the pause persists more than a few seconds. During the sinus pause, the P wave, QRS complex and PR and QRS intervals are all absent. P:QRS ratio is 1:1 and the rhythm is irregular. The pulse rate may vary widely, usually 60 to 100. Patients frequently complain of dizziness or syncope.

First-degree AV block

First degree AV block occurs when the atrial impulses are conducted through the AV node to the ventricles at a rate that is slower than normal. While the P and QRS are usually normal, the PR interval is >0.20 seconds, and the P:QRS ratio is 1:1. A narrow QRS complex indicates a conduction abnormality only in the AV node, but a widened QRS indicates associated damage to the bundle branches as well. Chronic first-degree block may be caused by fibrosis/sclerosis of the conduction system related to coronary artery disease, valvular disease, and cardiac myopathies and carries little morbidity. Acute first-degree block, on the other hand, is of much more concern and may be related to digoxin toxicity, β-blockers, amiodarone, myocardial infarction, hyperkalemia, or edema related to valvular surgery.

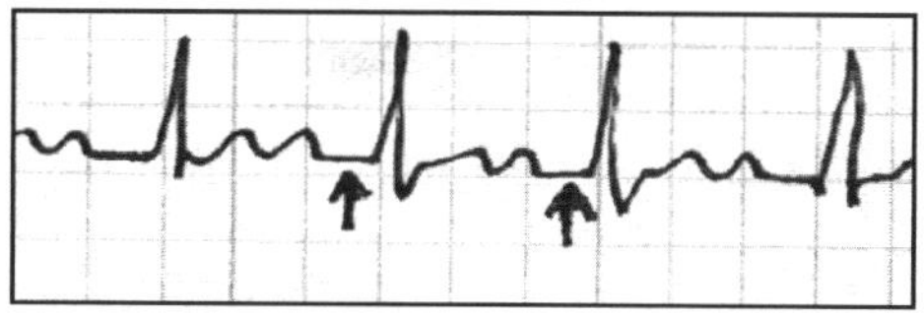

Second-degree AV block, type I

Second-degree AV block occurs when some of the atrial beats are blocked. Second-degree AV block is further subdivided according to the patterns of block: **Mobitz type I block (Wenckebach):** Each atrial impulse in a group of beats is conducted at a lengthened interval until one fails to conduct (the PR interval progressively increases), so there are more P waves than QRS, but the QRS complex is usually of normal shape and duration. The sinus node functions at a regular rate, so the P-P interval is regular, but the R-R interval usually shortens with each impulse. The P:QRS ratio varies, such as 3:2, 4:3, 5:4. This type of block by itself usually does not cause significant morbidity unless associated with inferior wall myocardial infarction.

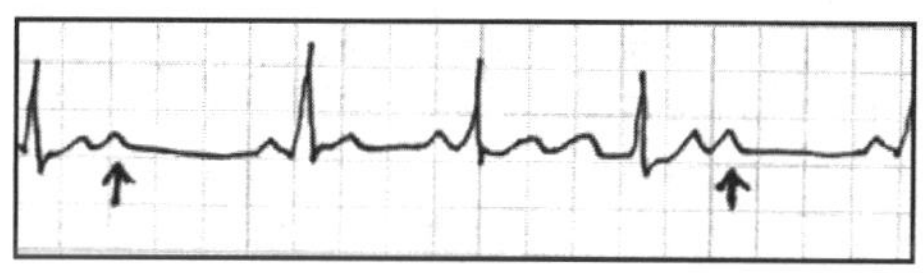

Second-degree AV block, type II, and 2:1 block

With **second-degree AV block, type II (Mobitz)**, only some of the atrial impulses are conducted unpredictably through the AV node to the ventricles, and the block always occurs below the AV node in the bundle of His, the bundle branches, or the Purkinje fibers. The PR intervals are the same if impulses are conducted, and QRS complex is usually widened. The P:QRS ratio varies 2:1, 3:1, and 4:1. Type II block is more dangerous than type I because it may progress to complete AV block and may produce Stokes-Adams syncope. Additionally, if the block is at the Purkinje fibers, there is no escape impulse. Usually a transcutaneous cardiac pacemaker and defibrillator should be at bedside. Symptoms may include chest pain if the heart block is precipitated by myocarditis or myocardial ischemia. **2:1 block:** Every other atrial impulse (P:QRS ratio of 2.1) is conducted through the AV node.

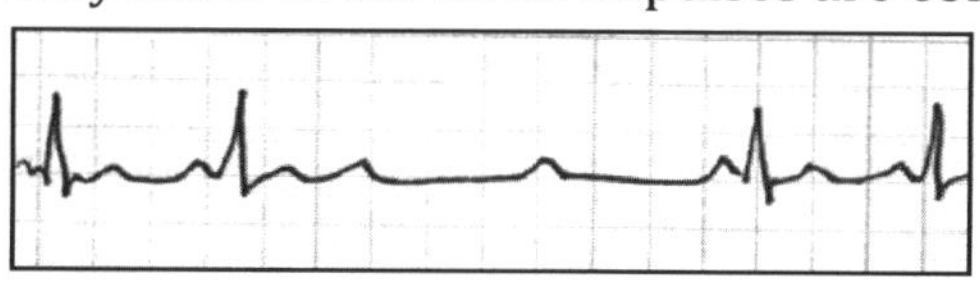

Third-degree AV block

With **third-degree AV block**, there are more P waves than QRS with no clear relationship between them and an atrial rate 2–3 times the pulse rate, so the PR interval is irregular. If the SA node malfunctions, the AV node fires at a lower rate, and if the AV node malfunctions, the pacemaker site in the ventricles takes over at a bradycardic rate; thus, with complete AV block, the heart still contracts, but often ineffectually. With this type of block, the atrial P (sinus rhythm or atrial fibrillation) and the ventricular QRS (ventricular escape rhythm) are stimulated by different impulses, so there is AV dissociation. The heart may compensate at rest but can't keep pace with exertion. The resultant bradycardia may cause congestive heart failure, fainting, or even sudden death, and usually conduction abnormalities slowly worsen. Symptoms include dyspnea, chest pain, and hypotension, which are treated with IV atropine. Transcutaneous pacing may be needed. Complete persistent AV block normally requires implanted pacemakers, usually dual chamber.

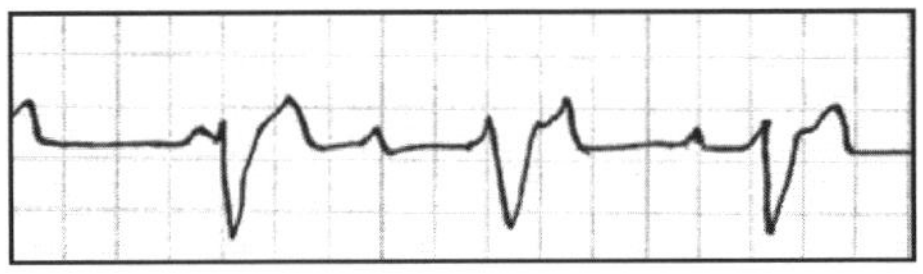

Discuss RBBB and LBBB

A **right bundle branch block** (RBBB) occurs when conduction is blocked in the right bundle branch that carries impulses from the Bundle of His to the ventricles. The impulse travels through the myocardium, but this causes a slight delay in contraction of the right ventricle. RBBB A left bundle branch block is characterized by normal P waves, but the QRS complex is widened and notched (rabbit-eared) although this may not be seen with minimal leads sometimes used in monitoring PR interval is normal or prolonged, and the QRS interval is > 0.12 seconds. P:QRS ratio remains 1:1 with regular rhythms, usually in the 60 to 100 range.

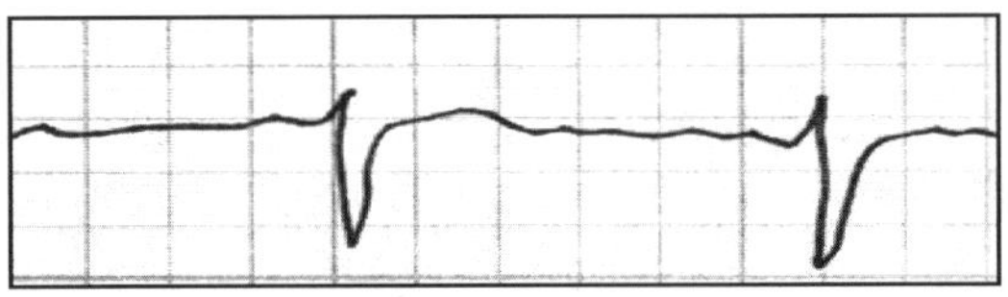

A **left bundle branch block** (LBBB) is characterized by normal P waves, but the QRS complex may be widened and notched (M-shaped) with interval of >0.12 seconds. The PR interval may be normal or prolonged. The P:QRS ratio is 1:1 and rhythm is regular, usually in the 60 to 100 range.

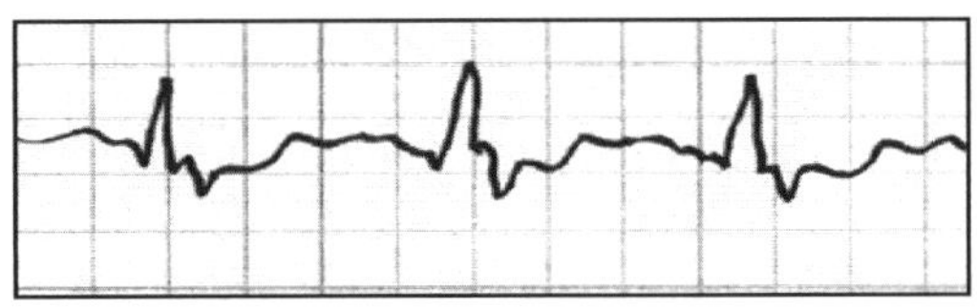

Heart failure symptoms

Heart failure symptoms vary widely depending upon the type and degree, the primary cause, and the child's age. Because of increased pressure in the lungs after birth, symptoms may be delayed in infants for the first week or two.

- **Infants** with left failure typically suffer respiratory distress with tachypnea, grunting respirations, sternal retraction, and rales, but the most common symptom is failure to thrive and difficulty eating, often leaving the child exhausted and sweaty. Those with right-sided failure may have more generalized edema of lower extremities, distended abdomen from ascites, hepatomegaly and jugular venous distension. Tachycardia and low cardiac output occurs with both types of heart failure resulting in sweating, pallor, and hypotension.
- **Older children** typically suffer from inability to tolerate activity or exercise, becoming short of breath on exertion. Appetite is often poor with weight loss.

- **In adolescents**, HF may be caused by the use of illicit drugs if there is no structural or acquired heart disease.

Congestive heart failure management

Management of heart failure (HF) in infants and children can be difficult. It is extremely important to establish the etiology and to treat the underlying cause. For infants with structural cardiac abnormalities, surgical repair may be needed to resolve the HF. There are some medical treatments that can relieve symptoms:

- **Diuretics**, such as furosemide (Lasix®), metolazone, or hydrochlorothiazide to reduce pulmonary and peripheral edema
- **Antihypertensives**, such as Captopril® or propranolol to decrease heart workload
- **Cardiac glycosides**, such as Lanoxin®, may relieve symptoms if above medicines are not successful.
- **High caloric feedings**, either by bottle or nasogastric feeding to provide sufficient nutrients
- **Oxygen** may be useful for some children with weak hearts.
- Restriction of activities to reduce stress on the heart
- **Dopamine or dobutamine** may be given to increase the contractibility of the heart.

Infective endocarditis

Infective endocarditis occurs when bacteria invade heart tissue or heart valves, usually in those with preexisting heart disorders. Risk factors include prosthetic heart valves, previous endocarditis, history of rheumatic fever or other disorder causing valve damage, congenital heart defects (ventricular or atrial septal defects), history of drug use, heart transplant recipient, and hypertrophic cardiomyopathy. Diagnosis is per blood cultures and positive echocardiogram.

Signs and symptoms	Treatment
Symptoms may vary widely and be nonspecific with low-grade symptoms persisting for >2 weeks and acute symptoms <2 weeks: Fever (present in most), chills, sweats Myalgia, arthralgia Fatigue and general malaise Headache Cough Confusion	Parenteral antimicrobial agents, depending on the pathogenic agent, usually for 4 to 8 weeks Prophylaxis is recommended for GU and GI procedures; for dental procedures, ONLY for those with prosthetic valves or other prosthetic material for heart repair, or history of or current heart disease.

Myocarditis

Myocarditis is inflammation of the cardiac myocardium (muscle tissue), usually triggered by a viral infection, such as the influenza virus, Coxsackie virus, and HIV. Myocarditis can also be caused by bacteria, fungi, or parasites. In some cases, it is also a complication of endocarditis. Myocarditis may also be triggered by chemotherapy drugs and some antibiotics. One problem with children is that the immune response against the invading organism may be overly aggressive, invading the heart muscle and producing toxins that damage cells and cause further damage to the heart muscle. Myocarditis can result in dilation of the heart, development of thrombi on the heart walls (known as mural thrombi), and infiltration of blood cells around the coronary vessels and between muscle fibers, causing further degeneration of the muscle tissue. The heart may become enlarged and weak, as the ability to pump blood is impaired, leading to congestive heart failure.

Diagnosis of myocarditis depends upon the clinical picture, as there is no test specific for myocarditis although a number of tests may be done to verify the clinical diagnosis:

- Chest radiograph may indicate cardiomegaly or pulmonary edema.
- EKG may show nonspecific changes.
- Echocardiogram may indicate cardiomegaly and demonstrate defects in functioning.
- Cardiac catheterization and cardiac biopsy will yield confirmation in 65% of cases, but not all of the heart muscle may be affected, so a negative finding does not rule out myocarditis.
- Viral cultures of nasopharynx and rectum may help to identify organism.
- Viral titers may increase as disease progresses.
- Polymerase chain reaction (PCR) of biopsy specimen may be most effective for diagnosis.

Treatment aims to meet hemodynamic needs and maintain tissue perfusion: Restriction of activities. Careful monitoring for heart failure and medical treatment as indicated (diuretics, digoxin, etc.). Oxygen as needed to maintain normal oxygen saturation. IV gamma globulin for acute stage

Pericarditis

Pericarditis is inflammation of the pericardial membrane that surrounds the heart. The outer fibrous pericardium is connective tissue that is continuous with the outer layers of the great vessels and serves to protect and anchor the heart. The inner serous pericardium has two layers separated with serous pericardial fluid to lubricate the heart and prevent friction. With pericarditis, the layers may become attached to each other (dry), or the serous fluid may be replaced by purulent material, calcifications, fibrinous material, or blood. Pericarditis is frequently associated with surgical repair of cardiac structural abnormalities, but it may also result from other systemic viral, bacterial, fungal, or parasitic infections or may be caused by direct trauma. Some chronic connective tissue disorders, such as lupus erythematosus, may also cause pericarditis. Pericarditis is often accompanied by fever, dysrhythmia, poor appetite, irritability, malaise, and sharp piercing chest pain.

Pericarditis is treated according to the cause and the type and extent of inflammation as well as the age, size, and condition of the child. Diagnostic procedures are similar to those for endocarditis and myocarditis. Treatment includes:

- Analgesics as indicated to control pain.
- Anti-inflammatory drugs, aspirin or ibuprofen, may be used to relieve discomfort and increase the rate of fluid reabsorption.
- Restriction of activity is necessary if cardiac function and output is impaired.
- Corticosteroids are used in some cases if there is no response to anti-inflammatory drugs.
- Surgical intervention may include pericardiocentesis, which is removing fluid from the pericardial sac in order to relieve increasing pressure and to diagnose the causative agent. In some cases, a small opening may be made into the pericardium to allow continuous drainage of exudate into the chest cavity. In severe cases, the outer layer of the pericardium may need to be removed if it is preventing functioning of the ventricles.

Aortic stenosis

Aortic stenosis is a stricture (narrowing) of the aortic valve that controls the flow of blood from the left ventricle, causing the left ventricular wall to thicken as it increases pressure to overcome the valvular resistance, increasing afterload, and increasing the need for blood supply from the coronary arteries. This condition may result from a birth defect or childhood rheumatic fever and tends to worsen over the years as the heart grows.

Symptoms	Treatment
Chest pain on exertion and intolerance of exercise. Heart murmur. Hypotension on exertion may be associated with sudden fainting. Sudden death can occur. Tachycardia with faint pulse. Poor feeding. Increased risk for bacterial endocarditis and coronary insufficiency. Increased mitral regurgitation and secondary pulmonary hypertension.	**Note:** Treatment in children may be done before symptoms develop because of the danger of sudden death. Balloon valvuloplasty to dilate valve non-surgically. Surgical repair of valve or replacement of valve, depending upon the extent of stricture.

Ventriculoperitoneal shunts

Ventriculoperitoneal shunts are inserted to treat hydrocephalus, relieving increased intracranial pressure from collection of excess CSF. The shunt creates a pathway to divert CSF. Shunts are usually comprised of a ventricular catheter (placed in the ventricles), a pump or reservoir (placed under the scalp), a one-way valve, and a distal catheter draining CSF into the peritoneum. **Shunt malfunction or failure** may relate to occlusion, sometimes because of infection, or damage to the shunt, such as breaking of catheters. Indications of shunt malfunction include indications of increasing ICP, such as headache, nausea, vomiting, alterations in mental status, lethargy, drowsiness, increasing head circumference, bulging of fontanels (in infants). With infection, fever, erythema, and induration along shunt tract, or indications of meningitis may be evident. Infection and pressure may be assessed by aspirating fluid from the reservoir. Infection requires immediate treatment with antibiotics. If the shunt is occluded or mechanically damaged, surgical revision or replacement is necessary.

Neurological

Brain tumors

Brain tumors in children can include astrocytoma, brain stem glioma, craniopharyngioma, ependymoma, ganglioglioma, medulloblastoma, oligodendroglioma, and optical nerve glioma. The most common age of onset is 3 to 12. Children may present with a wide range of symptoms. Signs and symptoms relate to the affected lobe and speed of growth:

- **Frontal:** Changes in personality and mood and hemiparesis
- **Temporal:** Lack of coordination, speech difficulty (slow, slurring), and memory loss
- **Parietal:** Sensory abnormalities, loss of fine motor skills and half-body awareness, difficulty writing
- **Cerebellum:** Lack of coordination and balance
- **Occipital:** Vision impairment, disturbances and visual hallucinations
- **Brain stem:** Facial pain, difficulty swallowing, cranial nerve abnormalities

As the tumor grows, a variety of symptoms may occur, including increasing intracranial pressure, hydrocephalus, compression of vasculature resulting in ischemia, focal neurological abnormalities, hemorrhage from invasion of vessels, and seizures. Pressure on the pituitary gland may result in inappropriate antidiuretic hormone or diabetes insipidus. Diagnosis is with MRI. Treatment includes surgery, radiation, and/or chemotherapy.

Partial seizures

Partial seizures are caused by an electrical impulse discharged to a localized area of the cerebral cortex, such as the frontal, temporal, or parietal lobes with seizure characteristics related to area of involvement. They may begin in a focal area and become generalized, often preceded by an aura.

- **Simple partial:** unilateral motor symptoms including somatosensory, psychic, and autonomic
- Aversive: eyes and head turned away from focal side
- Sylvan (usually during sleep): tonic-clonic movements of the face, salivation, and arrested speech
- **Special sensory:** various sensations (numbness, tingling, prickling, or pain) spreading from one area. May include visual sensations, posturing or hypertonia. Rare <8 years.
- **Complex (psychomotor):** No loss of consciousness, but altered consciousness and nonresponsive with amnesia. May involve complex sensorium with bad tastes, auditory or visual hallucinations, feeing of déjà vu, strong fear. May carry out repetitive activities, such as walking, running, smacking lips, chewing, or drawling. Rarely aggressive. Seizure usually followed by prolonged drowsiness and confusion. Occurs 3 through adolescence.

Generalized seizures

Generalized seizures lack a focal onset and appear to involve both hemispheres, usually presenting with loss of consciousness and no preceding aura.

- **Tonic-clonic** (Grand Mal): Occurs without warning
- **Tonic period** (10–30 seconds): Eyes roll upward with loss of consciousness, arms flexed, stiffen in symmetric tonic contraction of body, apneic with cyanosis and salivating.
- **Clonic period** (10 seconds to 30 minutes, but usually 30 seconds): Violent rhythmic jerking with contraction and relaxation. May be incontinent of urine and feces. Contractions slow and then stop.
- **Absence (Petit Mal):** Onset between 4–12 and usually ends in puberty. Onset is abrupt with brief loss of consciousness for 5–10 seconds and slight loss of muscle tone but often appears to be daydreaming. May include lip smacking or eye twitching.

Following seizures, there may be confusion, disorientation, and impairment of motor activity, speech and vision for several hours. May involve headache, nausea, and vomiting. Child often falls asleep and awakens conscious.

Generalized seizures

Generalized seizures include:

- **Atonic and akinetic (drop attacks):** Onset 2–5 years. Sudden loss of muscle tone and control of posture causes child to fall violently to the floor. Loss of consciousness may be momentary. May recur frequently during the daytime, and child may have serious injuries from falls.
- **Myoclonic seizures:** Sudden brief muscle contractures, single or repetitively. May be symmetric. No loss of consciousness, and may occur independently or associated with other types of seizures.

- **Infantile myoclonus (spasm):** Occurs ≤ 8 months, more commonly in males. Series of sudden short, symmetric muscle contractions with head flexed, arms extended, and knees drawn up OR extensor spasms of trunk and head nodding. May occur repeatedly during day. May have "lightning," very short momentary contraction of body. May lose consciousness and eyes may roll upward. Often causes cognitive impairment.

Febrile seizure

Febrile seizure is a generalized seizure associated with fever (usually >38.8ºC, 101.8º F) from any type of infection (URI, urinary) but without intracranial infection or other cause, occurring between 6 months and 5 years of age. Careful clinical examination must be conducted to rule out more serious disorders. Laboratory tests are conducted in relation to symptoms. Lumbar puncture is not usually indicated unless intracranial infection is suspected. Seizures usually last <15 minutes and are without subsequent neurological deficit. Treatment includes:

- Fever control: Acetaminophen 10–15mg/kg every 4 hours OR ibuprofen 10mg/kg every 6–8 hours
- Tepid water bath (NOT alcohol)
- Repeat seizures or history of febrile seizures: Phenobarbital 15mg/kg IV and 4–6mg/kg each day until improvement
- Anti-epileptic drugs (AEDs) (usually not advised unless seizures are complex, child is <6 months, or there is a pre-existing neurological disorder): Diazepam 0.2–0.5mg/kg every 8 hours during fever (may cause lethargy)

Status epilepticus

Status epilepticus (SE) is usually generalized tonic-clonic seizures that are characterized by a series of seizures with intervening time too short for regaining of consciousness. The constant assault and periods of apnea can lead to exhaustion, respiratory failure with hypoxemia and hypercapnia, cardiac failure, and death.

Causes	Treatment
Uncontrolled epilepsy or noncompliance with anticonvulsants. Infections, such as encephalitis. Encephalopathy or stroke. Drug toxicity (isoniazid). Brain trauma. Neoplasms. Metabolic disorders.	Anticonvulsants usually beginning with fast-acting benzodiazepine (Ativan®), often in steps, with administration of medication every 5 minutes until seizures subside. If cause is undetermined, acyclovir and ceftriaxone may be administered. If there is no response to the first 2 doses of anticonvulsants (refractory SE), rapid sequence intubation (RSI), which involves sedation and paralytic anesthesia, may be done while therapy continues. Combining phenobarbital and benzodiazepine can cause apnea, so intubation may be necessary. Phenytoin and phenobarbital are given.

West Nile virus

West Nile virus is an RNA virus, spread by infected mosquitoes. Infection has been traced to donor organs, blood transfusions, and breast milk, although the blood supply has been monitored for WNV since 2003. While WNV is more common in adults, especially the elderly, it can affect infants and children. Infected children show symptoms more readily than adults. The incubation period ranges from 2–14 days. There are 3 types of infection:

- **Viremia:** 80%, infection but no symptoms.
- **Mild:** 20% (West Nile fever), characterized by fever, malaise, lymphadenopathy, headache, rash, nausea, and vomiting. The acute stage is usually is self-limiting within a few days, but

symptoms can persist for weeks, including muscular weakness, fatigue, concentration problems, fever, and headache. About 30% require hospitalization.

- **Severe:** <1%, severe neurological symptoms with meningitis and associated symptoms being the most common in children and young adults.

There is no treatment for the virus. Treatment is supportive during illness and preventive (insect repellant).

Bacterial meningitis

Bacterial meningitis may be caused by a wide range of pathogenic organisms, with the predominant agents varying with the child's age:

- ≤1 month: Escherichia coli, Group B streptococci, Listeria monocytogenes, and Neisseria meningitidis.
- 1–2 months: Group B streptococci.
- >2 months: Streptococcus pneumoniae, Neisseria meningitidis. Unvaccinated (Hib vaccine) children are at risk for Haemophilus influenzae.

Bacterial infections usually arise from distant infections although they can enter the CNS from surgical wounds, invasive devices, nasal colonization, or penetrating trauma. The infective process includes inflammation, exudates, white blood cell accumulation, and tissue damage with the brain showing evidence of hyperemia and edema. Purulent exudate covers the brain and invades and blocks the ventricles, obstructing CSF and leading to increased intracranial pressure. Since antibodies specific to bacteria don't cross the blood/brain barrier, the body's ability to fight the infection is very poor. Diagnosis is usually based on lumbar puncture examination of cerebrospinal fluid and symptoms.

Bacterial meningitis may manifest differently, depending upon the age of the child.

- **Neonates:** Signs may be very nonspecific, such as weight loss, hypo- or hyperthermia, jaundice, irritability, lethargy, irregular respirations with periods of apnea. More specific signs may include increasing signs of illness, difficulty feeding with loss of suck reflex, hypotonia, weak cry, seizures, and bulging fontanels (may be a late sign). Nuchal rigidity does not usually occur with neonates.
- **Infants and young children:** Classic symptoms usually don't appear until ≥2 years. Signs may include fever, poor feeding, vomiting, irritability, and bulging fontanel. Nuchal rigidity in some children.
- **Older children and adolescents:** Abrupt onset, including fever, chills, headache, and alterations of consciousness with seizures, agitation, and irritability. May have photophobia, hallucinations, aggressive behavior or stupor and lapse into coma. Nuchal rigidity progressing to opisthotonos. Reflexes are variable but positive Kernig and Brudzinski signs. Signs may relate to particular bacteria, such as rashes, sore joints, or draining ear.

Patients with **bacterial meningitis** may exhibit signs to help support the diagnosis. While the following are not universally present, they are specific to meningitis and are rarely positive with other disorders.

Kernig's sign: Flex each hip and then try to straighten the knee while the hip is flexed. Spasm of the hamstrings makes this painful and difficult with meningitis.

Brudzinski sign: With the child lying supine, flex the neck by pulling head toward chest. The neck stiffness causes the hips and knees to pull up into a flexed position with meningitis.

Jolt accentuation maneuver (used if nuchal rigidity is not present): Ask child to rapidly move his/her head from side to side horizontally. Increase in headache is positive for meningitis.

Ischemic strokes

Ischemic strokes occur when an area of the brain is deprived of oxygen after an artery is occluded because of thrombus formation (as with sickle cell anemia or lupus erythematosus) or embolus (as with cardiac abnormalities or surgery). Medical management is similar to that for adults.

- **Thrombolytics**, such as tPA, which is produced by recombinant DNA and used to dissolve fibrin clots, should be initiated within 3 hours. It is given intravenously (0.5 mg/kg) with 10% injected as an initial bolus and the rest over the next hour; increases risk of bleeding.
- **Anticoagulation:** Heparin may be given with a loading dose of 75 U/kg followed by 20 U/kg/hr (>1 year) or 28 U/kg/hr (<1 yr) to APTT of 60–85 sec. Aspirin may be used with embolism.
- **Antihypertensives** to reduce hypertension
- **Cooling** to reduce hyperthermia
- **Osmotic diuretics** (mannitol), hypertonic saline, loop diuretics (Lasix®), and/or corticosteroids (dexamethasone) to reduce cerebral edema and intracranial pressure
- **Stool softeners** to prevent constipation
- Monitoring and treating hyperglycemia

Hemorrhagic strokes

Hemorrhagic strokes result from a ruptured cerebral artery, causing not only lack of oxygen and nutrients but also edema that causes widespread pressure and damage.

Intracerebral is bleeding into the substance of the brain from an artery in the central lobes, basal ganglia, pons, or cerebellum. Intracerebral hemorrhage usually results from hypertension, brain tumors, anticoagulation therapy, or some illicit drugs, such as crack and cocaine. Onset is often sudden and may cause death.

Intracranial aneurysm occurs when a ballooning cerebral artery ruptures, most commonly at the Circle of Willis.

Arteriovenous malformation (AVM) is a tangle of dilated arteries and veins without a capillary bed. This is a congenital abnormality. Rupture of AVMs is a cause of stroke, most common in young adults.

Subarachnoid hemorrhage is bleeding
in the space between the meninges and brain, resulting from aneurysm, AVM, or trauma. This type of hemorrhage compresses brain tissue.

Stroke symptoms

Strokes most commonly occur in the right or left hemisphere, but the exact location and the extent of brain damage affects the type of presenting symptoms. If the frontal area of either side is involved, there tend to be memory and learning deficits. Some symptoms are common to specific areas and help to identify the area involved, depending on the age of the child.

- **Right hemisphere:** This results in left paralysis or paresis and a left visual field deficit that may cause spatial and perceptual disturbances so that people may have difficulty judging distance. Fine motor skills may be impacted, resulting in trouble dressing or handling tools. Children may become impulsive and exhibit poor judgment, often denying impairment. Left-sided neglect (lack of perception of things on the left side) may occur. Depression is common as well as short-term memory loss and difficulty following directions. Language skills usually remain intact.
- **Left hemisphere:** This results in right paralysis or paresis and a right visual field defect. Depression is common, and children often exhibit slow, cautious behavior, requiring repeated instruction and reinforcement for simple tasks. Short-term memory loss and difficulty learning new material or understanding generalizations is common. Difficulty with mathematics, reading, writing, and reasoning may occur. Aphasia (expressive, receptive, or global) is common.
- **Brain stem:** Because the brain stem controls respiration and cardiac function, a brain attack frequently causes death, but those who survive may have a number of problems, including respiratory and cardiac abnormalities. Strokes may involve motor or sensory impairment or both.
- **Cerebellum:** This area controls balance and coordination. Strokes in the cerebellum are rare but may result in ataxia, nausea and vomiting, headaches, dizziness, or vertigo.

Migraine and tension headaches

Headaches are common in children and usually benign. About 3% of children develop migraine headaches before age 7 and up to 23% by age 11 or older, and many experience tension headaches. Sudden onset of headache, persistent or severe headache may indicate a pathological condition, such as increased intracranial pressure or tumor, so headaches should be evaluated carefully.

Type	Symptoms	Treatment
Migraine	Unilateral or bilateral, moderate to severe throbbing pain persisting ≤72 hours and sometimes preceded by visual or motor aura. Co-morbidities include nausea, vomiting, photophobia, or phonophobia. Young children may exhibit head banging, irritability, general malaise, and head holding.	NSAIDs, acetaminophen. Relaxation techniques. Biofeedback. Adolescents: sumatriptan nasal spray. Identifying and eliminating triggers, such as caffeine, foods, or additives.
Tension	Dull, aching, mild to moderate bilateral constricting pain about head, neck, and sometimes shoulders persisting hours or days. Pain unrelated to physical activity.	NSAIDs, acetaminophen. Ice pack. Rest. Relaxation techniques.

Rebound and sinus or dental-related headaches

Type	Symptoms	Treatment
Rebound (from excess medication use)	Vary but may be bilateral or unilateral in frontal area with frequency increasing with increased medication use. Tend to occur at least 5 times weekly or 15 times per month.	Withdrawal of medications (NSAIDs, acetaminophen, other drugs). Substitution with other drugs if headaches persist. Clonidine for withdrawal symptoms if necessary
Sinus- or dental-related	Dull constant pain and pressure over affected areas of sinus or dental abscess. Fever. Changing head position may vary pain.	NSAIDs, acetaminophen. Antibiotics. Application of cold or heat. Surgical drainage of sinus may be indicated for severe infection. Dental treatment as needed.

Hydrocephalus

Symptoms of hydrocephalus depend on the age of onset. In early infancy, before closure of cranial sutures, head enlargement is the most common presentation, but in older children with less elasticity in the skull, neurological symptoms usually relate to increasing pressure on structures of the brain.

Early infancy: Bulging, non-pulsating fontanels (usually anterior) usually with increasing head circumference, dilated scalp veins, separating sutures, and positive Macewen sign (resonance on tapping near the frontal-temporal-parietal juncture).

Later signs: Enlargement of frontal area with depressed eyes, setting sun sign (sclera evident above iris), and pupils sluggish and unequally reactive.

Throughout infancy: Increased irritability, lethargy, high-pitched crying, delayed responses, change in level of consciousness, opisthotonos, spasticity, difficulty feeding, and cardiopulmonary compromise.

Childhood (related to increased intracranial pressure): Headache relieved by vomiting, papilledema, strabismus, ataxia, irritability, lethargy, confusion, and difficulty communicating.

Hydrocephalus is diagnosed through CT and MRI, which help to determine the cause. Treatment may vary somewhat depending upon the underlying disorder, which may require specific treatment. For example, if obstruction is caused by a tumor, surgical excision to directly remove the obstruction is required. Generally, however, most hydrocephalus is treated with shunts.

Ventricular-peritoneal shunt: This procedure is the most common and consists of placement of a ventricular catheter directly into the ventricles (usually lateral) at one end with the other end in the peritoneal area to drain away excess CSF. There is a one-way valve near the proximal end that prevents backflow but opens when pressure rises to drain fluid. In some cases the distal end drains into the right atrium. Post-op management includes monitoring VS, oxygen saturation, and neurological status for indications of increasing ICP.

Third ventriculostomy: A small opening is made in the base of the third ventricle so CSF can bypass an obstruction. This procedure is not common and is done with a small endoscope.

Arteriovenous malformation

Arteriovenous malformation (AVM) is a congenital abnormality within the brain consisting of a tangle of dilated arteries and veins without a capillary bed. AVMs can occur anywhere in the brain and may cause no significant problems. Usually the AVM is "fed" by one or more cerebral arteries, which enlarge over time, shunting more blood through the AVM. The veins also enlarge in response to increased arterial blood flow because of the lack of a capillary bridge between the two. Because vein walls are thinner and lack the muscle layer of an artery, the veins tend to rupture as the AVM becomes larger, causing a subarachnoid hemorrhage. Chronic ischemia that may be related to the AVM can result in cerebral atrophy. Sometimes small leaks, usually accompanied by headache and nausea and vomiting, may occur before rupture. AVMs may cause a wide range of neurological symptoms, including changes in mentation, dizziness, sensory abnormalities, confusion, increasing ICP, and dementia. Treatment includes:

Supportive management of symptoms
Surgical repair or focused irradiation (definitive treatments)

Gastrointestinal

Bowel obstructions

Bowel obstruction occurs when there is a mechanical obstruction of the passage of intestinal contents because of constriction of the lumen, occlusion of the lumen, or lack of muscular contractions (paralytic ileus). Obstruction may be caused by congenital or acquired abnormalities/disorders. Treatment depends on cause and includes barium enema and surgical repair.

Small bowel obstructions	**Large bowel obstructions**
Duodenal atresia Malrotation and volvulus Jejunoileal atresia Meconium ileus Meconium peritonitis	Hirschsprung disease Anorectal malformations Meconium plug syndrome
Symptoms of bowel obstructions	
Abdominal pain and distention Abdominal rigidity Vomiting and dehydration Diminished or no bowel sounds Severe constipation (obstipation) Respiratory distress from diaphragm pushing against pleural cavity Shock as plasma volume diminishes and electrolytes enter intestines from bloodstream Sepsis as bacteria proliferates in bowel and invade bloodstream	

Hirschsprung disease

Hirschsprung disease (congenital aganglionic megacolon) is failure of ganglion nerve cells to migrate to part of the bowel (usually the distal colon), so that part of the bowel lacks enervation and peristalsis, causing stool to accumulate and leading to distention and megacolon. There is a genetic predisposition to the disease that affects more males than females and is associated with trisomy 21 (Down syndrome). Symptoms include:

Neonatal diagnosis	Infancy diagnosis	Childhood diagnosis
Failure to pass meconium in 24–48 hours. Poor feeding. Bilious vomitus. Abdominal distention.	Chronic constipation. Failure to thrive. Periods of diarrhea and vomiting. Loud gurgling bowel sounds. (With infection) Severe enterocolitis with watery diarrhea fever, hypotension.	Chronic constipation with ribbon-like stools. Abdominal distention with visible peristalsis and palpable fecal abdominal mass. Poorly nourished. Anemia.

Treatment includes: Resection of aganglionic section and colorectal anastomosis. There are a number of procedures (Swenson, Duhamel, and Soave) but recently laparoscopic or trans-anal minimally invasive approaches have proven successful.

Intussusception

Intussusception is a telescoping of one portion of the intestine into another, usually at the ileocecal valve, causing an obstruction. As the walls of the intestine come in contact, inflammation and edema cause decreased perfusion, which can result in infarction with peritonitis and death. Fecal material cannot move past the obstruction. It is most common between 3–12 months but can occur until 6 years and may relate to viral infections.

Symptoms	Treatment
"Currant jelly stool" composed of blood and mucous (occurs with 60%). Sudden acute episodes of severe abdominal pain during which child pulls knees to chest. Vomiting. Lethargy and weakness. Distended abdomen, painful to palpation. Sausage-shaped mass in RUQ of abdomen. Progressive fever and prostration if peritonitis occurs.	Barium or air enema to diagnose and apply pressure that may resolve the intussusception. Surgical repair if there is shock, peritonitis, intestinal perforation, or failure to resolve with barium/air enema.

Adhesions

Adhesions are fibrous bands that cause intestinal loops to adhere to areas within the abdomen that heal slowly or scar after surgery. These bands can loop around the intestines and cause them to kink or bind them to other internal organs, sometimes resulting in partial or complete intestinal obstruction. Adhesions can occur in children who have had abdominal surgery or abdominal radiation treatments or may be congenital. Adhesions may increase in size over time and become more constrictive. Long-term sequelae includc infertility in adulthood (females). Symptoms, usually general abdominal discomfort, may be minimal unless obstruction occurs, at which time pain and distention becomes acute. Diagnosis is often made through exploratory surgery, as adhesions are not evident on x-ray or ultrasound. Partial obstructions may be treated with dietary modifications (liquid/low residue), although severe or complete obstructions require surgical repair.

Ulcerative colitis

Ulcerative colitis is superficial inflammation of mucosa of colon and rectum, causing ulcerations in the areas where inflammation has destroyed cells. These ulcerations, ranging from pinpoint to extensive, may bleed and produce purulent material. The mucosa of the bowel becomes swollen, erythematous, and granular. Onset is usually between ages 15 and 30, and there is a genetic component. Ulcerative colitis may affect only the rectum (ulcerative proctitis), the entire colon (pancolitis), or only the left colon (limited or distal colitis).

Signs and symptoms	Treatment
Abdominal pain may be absent or mild unless severe disease. Bloody diarrhea/rectal bleeding in absence of infection may result in anemia and fluid and electrolyte depletion. Diarrhea is more frequent as colonic involvement increases. Fecal urgency and tenesmus may occur. Anorexia resulting in weight loss, fatigue. Systemic disorders with eye inflammation, arthritis, liver disease, and osteoporosis as immune system triggers generalized inflammation.	Aminosalicylates. Steroids. Immunomodulatory agents. Antispasmodics. Iron supplementation. High protein diet with decreased fiber.

Crohn's disease

Crohn's disease manifests with inflammation of the GI system. Inflammation is transmural (often leading to intestinal stenosis and fistulas), focal, and discontinuous with aphthous ulcerations progressing to linear and irregularly shaped ulcerations. Granulomas may be present. Common sites of inflammation are the terminal ileum and cecum. Condition is usually chronic, but an acute flare-up may mimic appendicitis. Children may have delayed development and stunted growth. There is a genetic component to the disease.

Signs and symptoms	Treatment
Perirectal abscess/fistula in advanced disease. Diarrhea usually present with colonic disease. May have nocturnal bowel movements, watery stools, and rectal hemorrhage. Anemia may develop with chronic bleeding. Abdominal pain most common in lower right quadrant, usually indicating transmural inflammation; may include postprandial pain and cramping. Nausea and vomiting (usually related to small intestine strictures). Weight loss (with small intestine involvement). Fever and night sweats	Corticosteroids and antibiotics for acute exacerbations. Immunomodulatory agents (cyclosporine, methotrexate). Antidiarrheals. Aminosalicylates.

Peptic ulcer disease

Peptic ulcer disease (PUD) includes both ulcerations of the duodenum and stomach. They may be primary (usually duodenal) or secondary (usually gastric). Gastric ulcers are commonly associated with cytomegalovirus and *Helicobacter pylori* infections in children. *H. pylori* infection is spread in the fecal-oral route from person to person or contaminated water and causes a chronic inflammation and ulcerations of the gastric mucosa. PUD is 2–3 times more common in males and is associated with poor economic status resulting in a crowded unhygienic environment although it can occur in other children. Usually others in the family have a history of ulcers as well. Symptoms include abdominal pain, nausea, vomiting, and GI bleeding in children <6 with epigastric and postprandial pain and indigestion in older children. Treatment includes:

- Antibiotics for *H. pylori*: amoxicillin, clarithromycin, metronidazole
- Proton pump inhibitors: lansoprazole or omeprazole
- Sucralfate
- Histamine-receptor antagonists: cimetidine, ranitidine, and famotidine

Electrolyte imbalances

Sodium (Na) regulates fluid volume, osmolality, acid-base balance, and activity in the muscles, nerves and myocardium. It is the primary cation (positive ion) in ECF, necessary to maintain ECF levels that are needed for tissue perfusion.

Normal value: Infant 133 to 144 mEq/L, Child 135–145 mEq/L

Hyponatremia: <133 to 135 mEq/L (critical value <120)

Hypernatremia: >145–146 mEq/L (critical value >160)

Hyponatremia	May result from inadequate sodium intake or excess loss (through diarrhea, vomiting, NG suctioning). It can occur as the result of illness, such as severe burns, fever, SIADH, and ketoacidosis. Symptoms vary: Irritability to lethargy and alterations in consciousness. Cerebral edema with seizures and coma. Dyspnea to respiratory failure. Treatment*:* Identify and treat underlying cause and provide Na replacement.
Hypernatremia	May result from renal disease, diabetes insipidus, and fluid depletion. Symptoms include irritability to lethargy to confusion to coma, seizures, flushing, muscle weakness and spasms, and thirst. Treatment includes identifying and treating underlying cause, monitoring Na levels carefully, and IV fluid replacement.

Potassium (K) is the primary electrolyte in ICF with about 98% inside cells and only 2% in ECF, although this small amount is important for neuromuscular activity. K influences activity of the skeletal and cardiac muscles. K level is dependent upon adequate renal functioning because 80% is excreted through the kidneys and 20% through the bowels and sweat:

Normal values: Infant 4.1 to 5.3 mEq/L, Child 3.4 to 4.7 mEq/L

Hypokalemia: <3.4 mEq/L (age dependent). Critical value: <2.5 mEq/L

Hypokalemia	Caused by loss of K through diarrhea, vomiting, gastric suction, diuresis, alkalosis, decreased K intake with starvation, and nephritis. Symptoms include: Lethargy and weakness Nausea and vomiting Paresthesias Dysrhythmias with EKG abnormalities: PVCs, flattened T waves Muscle cramps with hyporeflexia Hypotension Tetany Treatment: Identify and treat underlying cause and replace K.

Hyperkalemia >5.5 mEq/L Critical value: >6.5 mEq/L	Caused by renal disease, adrenal insufficiency, metabolic acidosis, severe dehydration, burns, hemolysis, and trauma. It rarely occurs without renal disease but may be induced by treatment (such as use of NSAIDs and potassium-sparing diuretics). Untreated renal failure results in reduced excretion. Those with Addison's disease and deficient adrenal hormones suffer sodium loss that results in potassium retention. The primary symptoms relate to the effect on the cardiac muscle: Ventricular arrhythmias with increasing changes in EKG leading to cardiac and respiratory arrest. Weakness with ascending paralysis and hyperreflexia. Diarrhea Increasing confusion. Treatment includes identifying underlying cause and discontinuing sources of increased K: Calcium gluconate to decrease cardiac effects. Sodium bicarbonate shifts K into the cells temporarily. Insulin and hypertonic dextrose shift K into the cells temporarily. Cation exchange resin (Kayexalate®) to decrease K. Peritoneal dialysis or hemodialysis

Hypocalcemia and hypercalcemia

More than 99% of **calcium (Ca)** is in the skeletal system with 1% in serum, but it is important for transmitting nerve impulses and regulating muscle contraction and relaxation, including the myocardium. Calcium activates enzymes that stimulate chemical reactions and has a role in coagulation of blood. **Normal values**: 11 days to 2 years: 9 to 11 mg/dL. 3 to 12 years: 8.8 to 10.8 mg/dL. 13 to 18 years: 8.4 to 10.2 mg/dL.

- **Hypocalcemia**: <8.4 mg/dL. Critical value: <7 mg/dL
- **Hypercalcemia**: Age-dependent. Critical value: >12 mg/dL

Hypocalcemia	May be caused by hypoparathyroidism and occurs after thyroid and parathyroid surgery, pancreatitis, renal failure, inadequate vitamin D intake, alkalosis, magnesium deficiency, and low serum albumin. **Symptoms** include: Tetany, tingling, seizures, altered mental status. Ventricular tachycardia. **Treatment**: Calcium replacement and vitamin D
Hypercalcemia	May be caused by acidosis, kidney disease, hyperparathyroidism, prolonged immobilization, and malignancies. Crisis carries a 50% mortality rate. **Symptoms** include: Increasing muscle weakness with hypotonicity. Anorexia, nausea, and vomiting. Constipation. Bradycardia and cardiac arrest. **Treatment**: Identify and treat underlying cause, loop diuretics, and IV fluids

Hypophosphatemia and hyperphosphatemia

Phosphorus, or phosphate (PO_4), is necessary for neuromuscular and red blood cell function, the maintenance of acid-base balance, and provides structure for teeth and bones. About 85% is in the bones, 14% in soft tissue, and <1% in ECF. Normal values:

1 to 3 years: 3.9 to 6.5 mg/dL	12 to 13 years: 3.3 to 5.4 mg/dL
4 to 6 years: 4.0 to 5.4 mg/dL	14 to 15 years: 2.9 to 5.4 mg/dL
7 to 11 years: 3.7 to 5.6 mg/dL	16 to 19 years: 2.8 to 4.6 mg/dL
Hypophosphatemia. Critical value: <1 mg/dL	Occurs with severe protein-calorie malnutrition, excess antacids with magnesium, calcium or albumin, hyperventilation, severe burns, and diabetic ketoacidosis. **Symptoms** include: Irritability, tremors, seizures to coma. Hemolytic anemia. Decreased myocardial function. Respiratory failure **Treatment**: Identify and treat underlying cause and replace phosphorus.
Hyperphosphatemia	Occurs with renal failure, hypoparathyroidism, excessive intake, neoplastic disease, diabetic ketoacidosis, muscle necrosis, and chemotherapy. **Symptoms** include: Tachycardia. Muscle cramping, hyperreflexia, and tetany. Nausea and diarrhea. **Treatment**: Identify and treat underlying cause, correct hypocalcemia, and provide antacids and dialysis.

Hypomagnesemia and hypermagnesemia

Magnesium (Mg) is the second most common intracellular electrolyte (after potassium) and activates many intracellular enzyme systems. Mg is important for carbohydrate and protein metabolism, neuromuscular function, and cardiovascular function, producing vasodilation and directly affecting the peripheral arterial system. **Normal values** (child): 1.7 to 2.1 mEq/L.
Hypomagnesemia: <1.7 mEq/L. Critical value: <1.2 mg/dL
Hypermagnesemia: >2.1 mEq/L. Critical value: >4.9 mg/dL

Hypomagnesemia	Occurs with chronic diarrhea, chronic renal disease, chronic pancreatitis, excess diuretic or laxative use, hyperthyroidism, hypoparathyroidism, severe burns, and diaphoresis. **Symptoms** include: Neuromuscular excitability/ tetany, Confusion, headaches and dizziness, seizure and coma. Tachycardia with ventricular arrhythmias. Respiratory depression. **Treatment**: Identify and treat underlying cause, provide magnesium replacement.
Hypermagnesemia	Occurs with renal failure or inadequate renal function, diabetic ketoacidosis, hypothyroidism, and Addison's disease. Symptoms include muscle weakness, seizures, and dysphagia with decreased gag reflex, tachycardia with hypotension. Treatment: Identify and treat underlying cause, IV hydration with calcium, and dialysis.

Esophageal atresia and tracheoesophageal fistula

Esophageal atresia often occurs with **tracheoesophageal fistula** (TEF). In esophageal atresia, the esophagus has a blind pouch and does not completely pass to the stomach. In TEF, an abnormal connection is present between the trachea and the esophagus. A congenital tracheoesophageal fistula (TEF) may be associated with genetic anomalies, such as trisomy 13, 18, or 21 and various other anomalies. TEF is often associated with polyhydramnios, as esophageal atresia prevents the fetus from swallowing amniotic fluid. Acquired TEF may be secondary to intubation trauma or neoplasms.

Symptoms	Treatment
Fine, white, frothy bubbles of mucous in the mouth and nose. Copious secretions, despite suctioning. Episodes of coughing, choking, and cyanosis, which worsen with feeding	Enteral feedings or gastrostomy feedings. Mechanical ventilation and a cuffed endotracheal tube (preventing reflux until child stabilizes enough for surgical repair). Maintaining cuff pressures <25 mm Hg (helps prevent traumatic TEF)

Failure to thrive

Failure to thrive (FTT) is a descriptive term for children who exhibit inadequate growth and development, usually measured by the child's being below the 5th percentile for weight (and sometimes height). Failure to thrive may relate to physical causes (such as renal disease or congenital heart disease), psychosocial factors (such as poverty, neglect), or idiopathic factors (unexplained). However, many issues may be involved other than just the parent-child relationship.

- **Income:** Inability to buy sufficient or nutritional food
- **Health beliefs:** Child subjected to extreme or fad diets (vegan, low fat) without ensuring proper nutrition
- **Lack of education:** Inadequate knowledge of proper nutritional requirements for children
- **Stress:** Illness, single-family home, divorce, lack of employment, incarceration
- **Psychosocial issues:** Postpartum depression, other mental illnesses, or Munchausen syndrome by proxy
- **Resistance to feeding:** History of NG feedings, cleft lip/palate, or esophageal atresia
- **Inadequate supply of milk:** Poor breastfeeding technique or poor milk supply

Failure to thrive (FTT) is diagnosed first by identifying children at risk because of their evidence of growth failure.
Diagnostic measures:
Weight/height percentile (5th percentile for weight indicative of FTT). Dietary intake history: Previous 24 hours and 3- to 5-day period. Evaluation of genetic factors: Family history, including heights/weights of parents. Identification of food allergies and food restrictions. Evaluation of meal behaviors/ practices. Lab tests as indicated to check for conditions such as anemia, parasites, and lead poisoning. Observation of family interactions, situation.

Management: Nutritional program to reverse evidence of malnutrition. Formula: Kcal per day = RDA for age in kcal/kg X ideal weight/actual weight. Vitamin and mineral supplements. Infants (young): Provide supplements to formula. Kcal per ounce of formula should not exceed 24. Toddlers: Provide high-caloric milk drink (PediaSure). Referrals to social workers, welfare, child protective services as indicated. Behavior modification related to meal times, eating habits interfering with nutrition. Family therapy as indicated. Family education. Structured supportive environment for feeding. Persistence in feeding and elimination of distractions. Slow introduction of new foods.

Common diet deficiencies

Common dietary deficiencies in infants and children	
Calcium	Calcium is essential for the growth and development of bones, but children, especially teenagers, are increasingly substituting fruit juice and sodas for milk. This can cause fractures and osteomalacia with eventual osteoporosis as an adult. Recommended daily intake for adolescents is 1500mg.
Folic acid	Intake is often low among teenagers, resulting in high rates of congenital abnormalities if they get pregnant. Cereals and breads are fortified with folic acid to combat this.
Iron	Newborns deplete their maternally supplied iron by about 4 months and may become anemic if breastfed without supplementary rice cereal. Formula is iron-fortified. Teenage girls are also often iron-deficient because of menses and poor dietary intake.
Vitamin D	Deficiencies are on the rise because of judicious use of sunscreen and protecting children from all sun exposure. Breast-fed infants may need vitamin D supplements.

Infant formulas

A wide variety of **infant formulas** are available, but the 3 primary types include:

- **Cow's milk-based formulas** (Enfamil®, Similac®, and Good Start®): Appropriate for most infants. These are enriched with various components, including vitamins, minerals, iron, tyrosine, phenylalanine, and carnitine.
- **Soy-based formulas** (Isomil®, Soyalac®, ProSobee®, Nursoy®): Appropriate for infants with primary lactose deficiency or galactosemia and those allergic to cow's milk-based formulas.
- **Therapeutic formulas** (Nutramigen®, Pregestimil®): Many preparations are available to meet special needs for infants with formula intolerance.

- **Pregestimil®** is a hypoallergenic formula specially designed for infants with malabsorption caused by gastrointestinal or hepatobiliary disease. It provides hydrolyzed (predigested) protein that is easier to digest. The majority of the fats are in the form of medium chain triglycerides (MCT). MCTs are easier to digest than other forms of fats.
- **Similac® PM 60/40** is a cow's milk-based formula that has a low phosphorus content and low renal solute load. It is designed for infants with impaired renal function or with hypocalcemia due to hyperphosphatemia. It has a whey-to-casein ratio of 60:40.
- **Nutramigen® LIPL** is a hypoallergenic formula designed for infants sensitive to the intact protein found in cow's milk-based formula. The proteins are hydrolyzed (digested) and easier to absorb. Cow's milk protein allergy is an indication for use of this formula. It contains docosahexaenoic (DHA) acid and arachidonic acid (ARA) that are also found in breast milk. DHA and ARA are omega 3 and 6 fatty acids that support normal brain, eye, and nerve development.

Formula may be purchased in ready-to-feed bottles or cans that require no preparation, liquid concentrate, or powder. Concentrate and powder require the addition of water, so a clean water supply and ability to measure correctly are necessary to avoid inadequate or unsafe nutrition. Babies who are bottle-fed with formula usually feed less frequently than those who are breastfed. Neonates usually take 2 to 3 ounces of formula every 3 to 4 hours. Neonates typically require approximately 2.5 ounces of formula for each pound (0.5 kg) of weight within each 24-hour period.

Obesity

Obesity in children and teenagers is increasing with 16–33% classified as overweight. While there is no clear agreement about weight standards for children, excess weight is having a profound effect on children's health. However, helping the child to lose weight can be difficult.

- Dieting is best approached as a healthier change in eating habits for the whole family so that the child does not eat differently from others.
- No more than 30% of nutrition should be fats.
- Carbohydrates should be complex rather than simple sugars, decreasing consumption of white flour and sugar.
- Healthy snacks, such as fruit, air-popped popcorn, and nonfat yogurt, should be provided with high-caloric snacks (chips, candy) not available.
- The child should eat 3 meals daily, served adequate but not large portions, and not be forced to "clean the plate."
- Television viewing or other sedentary activities should be progressively limited over time and exercise activities encouraged.

Genitourinary and Reproductive

Urethral strictures

Urethral strictures are rare in females because of the short length of the urethra but may occur in males as the result of congenital abnormality, mechanical injury (catheter, cystoscopy), prior surgical repairs (such as for hypospadias), trauma, or infection. Symptoms include penile edema, bladder distention, splaying or spraying urination, frequency, urgency, lower abdominal pain, and inability to urinate. Initial treatment may include insertion of catheter (urethral, suprapubic) to provide urinary drainage if obstruction is resulting in distention. If infection is present, antibiotics are indicated. Diagnostic tests include ultrasound, retrograde urethrogram, antegrade cystourethrogram, and cystourethrogram. A child with urethral strictures needs referral to a pediatric urologist for evaluation and treatment, which can include dilation and/or surgical or laser repair. Urethral strictures often recur, especially if treatment tears or cuts through strictures as this may cause more scarring.

Ovarian cyst

Ovarian cysts can grow within or on the ovaries. Functional: follicular cyst usually resolves in 1–3 months; corpus luteum usually resolves in a few weeks but cyst may grow to 4 inches, causing torsion and pain. Cystadenoma form on exterior of ovary and may enlarge and cause pain. Endometrioma attaches to ovaries and cause pain during menses and sexual activity. Dermoid cyst may enlarge and cause pain. Polycystic ovaries may have multiple cysts.

Diagnostic studies include pregnancy test to rule out ectopic pregnancy and ultrasound with Doppler flow. Ovarian cysts may cause problems if they rupture or hemorrhage and if they twist or become infected.

Signs and symptoms	Treatment
Hypotension and hypovolemia if hemorrhage occurs Pain (often acute) and tenderness in lower abdomen on affected side and/or lower back pain. Dysuria Weight gain	Note: Treatment depends upon the type of cyst and complications: Emergency surgery for torsion Antibiotics for infection Hormone therapy may be useful for endometrioma.

Cystitis

Urinary tract infections, such as cystitis, are common. *Escherichia coli* is the usual causative organism in pediatrics. UTIs may indicate GU abnormalities in children. UTIs are more common in girls than boys after the first year.

Signs and symptoms	Treatment
Changes in character of urine: *Appearance:* The urine may become cloudy from mucus or purulent material. Hematuria may be present. *Color:* Urine usually becomes concentrated and may be dark yellow/orange or brownish in color. *Odor*: Urine may have a very strong or foul odor.*Output:* Urinary output may decrease markedly. *Pain*: There may be lower back or flank pain from inflammation of the kidneys. *Systemic*: Fever, chills, headache, and general malaise often accompany urine infections. Some people suffer lack of appetite as well as nausea and vomiting. Fever usually indicates that the infection has affected the kidneys. Children may develop incontinence or loose stools and cry excessively.	Increased fluids. Acetaminophen. Antibiotics for 3 to 4 days.

Pyelonephritis

Pyelonephritis is a potentially organ-damaging bacterial infection of the parenchyma of the kidney. Pyelonephritis can result in abscess formation, sepsis, and kidney failure. Pyelonephritis is especially dangerous for children who are immunocompromised or diabetic. Most infections in children are caused by *Escherichia coli* or *Enterococcus faecalis*. Adolescent females often exhibit symptoms more associated with lower urinary infection, so the condition may be overlooked. Patients may require hospitalization or careful follow-up. Diagnostic studies include urinalysis, blood and urine cultures.

Signs and symptoms	Treatment
Dysuria and frequency, hematuria, flank and/or low back pain. Fever and chills. Costovertebral angle tenderness. Change in feeding habits (infants).	Analgesia. Antipyretics. Intravenous fluids. Antibiotics: Started initially but may be changed based on cultures. IV ceftriaxone with fluoroquinolone orally for 7–10 days Fluoroquinolone orally for 7–10 days

Acute renal failure

Acute renal failure is an abrupt and almost complete failure of kidney function with decreased glomerular filtration rate (GFR), occurring over a period of hours/days. It most commonly occurs in hospitalized patients but may occur in others as well. The BUN increases and nitrogenous wastes are retained (azotemia). There are 3 primary categories, related to cause:

- **Prerenal disorders**, such as myocardial infarction, heart failure, sepsis, anaphylaxis, and hemorrhage, result in hypoperfusion of the kidney and decreased GFR.

- **Intrarenal disorders** include burns, trauma, infection, transfusion reactions, and nephrotoxic agents that cause damage to glomeruli or kidney tubules, such as acute tubular necrosis. Burns and crush trauma injuries release myoglobin and hemoglobin from tissues, causing renal toxicity and/or ischemia. With transfusion reactions, hemolysis occurs, and the broken-down hemoglobin concentrates and precipitates in tubules. Medications, such as NSAIDs and ACE inhibitors may interfere with kidney function and cause hypoperfusion and ischemia.
- **Postrenal disorders** involve distal obstruction that increases pressure in tubules and decreases GFR.

Acute tubular necrosis

Acute tubular necrosis (ATN) occurs when a hypoxic condition causes renal ischemia that damages tubular cells of the glomeruli so they are unable to adequately filter the urine, leading to acute renal failure. Causes include hypotension, hyperbilirubinemia, sepsis, surgery (especially cardiac or vascular), and birth complications. ATN may result from nephrotoxic injury related to obstruction or drugs, such as chemotherapy, acyclovir, and antibiotics, such as sulfonamides and streptomycin. Symptoms may be nonspecific initially and can include life-threatening complications.

Symptoms	**Treatment**
Lethargy. Nausea and vomiting. Hypovolemia with low cardiac output and generalized vasodilation. Fluid and electrolyte imbalance leading to hypertension, CNS abnormalities, metabolic acidosis, arrhythmias, edema, and congestive heart failure. Uremia leading to destruction of platelets and bleeding, neurological deficits, and disseminated intravascular coagulopathy (DIC). Infections can include pericarditis and sepsis.	Identifying and treating underlying cause. Supportive care. Loop diuretics (in some cases), such as Lasix®. Antibiotics for infection. Discontinuation of nephrotoxic agents. Dopamine (low dose) to increase renal circulation. Kidney dialysis. Restricting potassium and phosphate.

End-stage renal disease

End-stage (chronic) renal disease (ESRD) occurs with chronic renal failure when the kidneys are unable to filter and excrete wastes, concentrate urine, and maintain electrolyte balance because of hypoxic conditions, kidney disease, or obstruction in the urinary tract. It results first in azotemia (increase in nitrogenous waste in the blood) and then in uremia (nitrogenous wastes cause toxic symptoms.) When >50% of the functional renal capacity is destroyed, the kidneys can no longer carry out necessary functions and progressive deterioration begins over months or years. Symptoms are often nonspecific in the beginning with loss of appetite and energy.

Symptoms and complications	Treatment
Weight loss. Headaches, muscle cramping, general malaise. Increased bruising and dry or itching skin. Increased BUN and creatinine. Sodium and fluid retention with edema. Hyperkalemia. Metabolic acidosis. Calcium and phosphorus depletion, resulting in altered bone metabolism, pain, and retarded growth. Anemia with decreased production of RBCs. Increased risk of infection. Uremic syndrome.	Supportive/symptomatic therapy. Dialysis and transplantation. Diet control: Low protein, salt, potassium, and phosphorus. Fluid limitations. Calcium and vitamin supplementation. Phosphate binders.

Renal dialysis

Renal dialysis is used primarily for those who have progressed from renal insufficiency to uremia with end-stage renal disease (ESRD). It may also be temporarily for acute conditions. Children can be maintained on dialysis, but there are many complications associated with dialysis so many children are considered for renal transplantation. There are a number of different approaches to dialysis.

Continuous renal replacement therapy (CRRT) circulates the blood by hydrostatic pressure through a semipermeable membrane. It is used in critical and emergency care and can be instituted quickly.

Continuous arteriovenous hemofiltration (CAVH) circulates blood from an artery (usually the femoral) to a hemofilter using only arterial pressure and not a blood pump. The filtered blood is then returned to the patient's venous system, often with added fluids to offset those lost. Only the fluid is filtered.

Continuous arteriovenous hemodialysis (CAVHD) is similar to CAVH except that dialysate circulates on one side of the semipermeable membrane to increase clearance of urea.

Continuous venovenous hemofiltration (CVVH) pumps blood through a double-lumen venous catheter to a hemofilter, which returns the blood to the patient in the same catheter. It provides continuous slow removal of fluid, is better tolerated with unstable patients, and doesn't require arterial access.

Continuous venovenous hemodialysis (CVVHD) is similar to CVVH but uses a dialysate to increase clearance of uremic toxins.

Peritoneal dialysis: An indwelling catheter is inserted surgically into the peritoneal cavity with a subcutaneous tunnel and a Dacron cuff to prevent infection. Sterile dialysate solution is slowly instilled through gravity, remains for a prescribed length of time, and is then drained and discarded.

Continuous ambulatory peritoneal dialysis: A series of exchange cycles are repeated 24 hours a day.
Continuous cyclic peritoneal dialysis: A prolonged period of retaining fluid occurs during the day with drainage at night.
Peritoneal dialysis may be used for those who want to be more independent, don't live near a dialysis center, or want fewer dietary restrictions.

Hemodialysis, the most common type of dialysis, is used for both short-term dialysis and long-term for those with ESRD. Treatments are usually done 3 times weekly for 3–4 hours or short daily dialysis with treatment either during the night or in short daily periods. Hemodialysis is often done for those who can't manage peritoneal dialysis or who live near a dialysis center, but it does interfere with work or school attendance and requires strict dietary and fluid restrictions between treatments. Short daily dialysis allows more independence, and increased costs may be offset by lower morbidity. A vascular access device, such as a catheter, fistula, or graft must be established for hemodialysis, and heparin is used to prevent clotting. With hemodialysis, blood is circulated outside of the body through a dialyzer (a synthetic semipermeable membrane), which filters the blood. There are many different types of dialyzers. High flux dialyzers use a highly permeable membrane that shortens the duration of treatment and decreases the need for heparin.

Gonorrhea

Gonorrhea is caused by *Neisseria gonorrhoeae* and should be suspected in sexually active adolescents with urinary infections. Symptoms include:

- **Males:** Dysuria and purulent discharge from the urethra, epididymitis, and prostatitis.

- **Females:** Many women are asymptomatic or may have lower abdominal pain, cystitis, or mucopurulent cervicitis, but untreated, it can result in PID and chronic pain.

Rectal infections are common in females and homosexual males. Untreated, gonorrhea can become a systemic infection, resulting in petechial or pustular skin lesions, arthralgias, tenosynovitis, fever and malaise, and septic arthritis. Diagnosis is by cervical or urethral culture or NAAT. Gram stains of urethral smears are more accurate for males than females. Cultures of multiple sites may be needed to confirm disseminated disease. Treatment includes:

- Cefixime 400 mg orally in one dose OR
- Ceftriaxone 125 mg IM in one dose OR
- Ciprofloxacin 500 mg orally in one dose OR
- Levofloxacin 250 mg orally in one dose.

Chlamydia

Chlamydia is a sexually transmitted disease (STD) caused by *Chlamydia trachomatis* and is often co-infected with gonorrhea. It may be transmitted by oral, anal, and vaginal sex. It is the most common STD in the United States. Diagnosis is most reliable from nucleic acid amplification test (NAAT) (AMPLICOR®, Probe TEC®).

Signs and symptoms	Treatment
Males: Urethritis, epididymitis, proctitis, or Reiter's syndrome (urethritis, rash, conjunctivitis). Many are asymptomatic. **Females:** Mild cervicitis with vaginal discharge and dysuria, but complications can lead to infertility and pelvic inflammatory disease (PID).	Azithromycin 1 g orally in one dose OR Doxycycline 100 mg orally twice daily for 1 week Avoidance of sexual contact for 1 week **Note:** Treatment of the infected person's sexual partner is very important to avoid reinfection after treatment.

Genital herpes

Genital herpes is caused by herpes simplex virus type 2 (HSV-2) (most common) or HSV-1. The virus infects mucous membranes or breaks in the skin, usually during sexual activity, and travels though the peripheral or autonomic nerve ending to the sensory or autonomic nerve ganglion where it rests dormant until it reactivates and descends to the original site of infection.

Signs and symptoms	Treatment
Initial infection: Burning, tingling Vesicular eruptions that ulcerate and then crust over Pain, fever, myalgia Dysuria Cervicitis with purulent vaginal discharge Reactivations: Similar to initial infection but usually less severe, and lesions usually heal in 1 to 2 weeks	Antiviral agents: Acyclovir, valacyclovir, and famciclovir Analgesia: Topical anesthetic (lidocaine) and analgesics (ASA, codeine) Supportive: Good genital hygiene and wearing loose cotton underwear reduces irritation Keep area dry (hair dryer on low setting) Sitz baths Preventive: Those infected should use barriers, such as condoms, during sexual activity to prevent transmission to others even when the virus is dormant

Human papillomavirus

Human papillomavirus (HPV) comprises >100 viruses. About 40 are sexually transmitted and invade mucosal tissue, causing genital warts, which are low risk for cancer, or changes in the mucosa, which can lead to cervical cancer. Most HPVs cause little or no symptoms, but they are very common, especially in those 15–25. Over 99% of cervical cancers are caused by HPV and 70% are related to HPVs 16 and 18. Vaccination is now recommended for all girls, ages ≥9–26 (usually given at ages 11–12 before sexual activity) and is also recommended for boys/men as well.

HPV vaccines	
Gardasil®	For prevention of HPV types 6, 11, 16, and 18. Effective for prevention of both cancer (cervical, vulvar, vaginal, and anal) and genital warts. This vaccine is administered in 3 separate doses: initial, 2 months later, and 6 months later.
Cervarix®	For prevention of HPV types 16 and 18. NOT effective for prevention of genital warts. This vaccine is administered in 3 separate doses: initial, 2 months later, and 6 months later.

Syphilis

Syphilis is caused by the spirochete *Treponema pallidum* and has increased in incidence over the last 10 years, associated with risk-taking behavior such as drug use. There are 3 phases to the disease, with an incubation period of about 3 weeks:

- **Primary:** Chancre (painless) in areas of sexual contact, persisting 3–6 weeks.
- **Secondary:** General flu-like symptoms (sore throat, fever, headaches) and red papular rash on trunk, flexor surfaces, palms, and soles, lymphadenopathy occur about 3–6 weeks after end of primary phase and eventually resolve.
- **Tertiary** (latent): Affects about 30% and includes CNS and cardiovascular symptoms 3–20 years after initial infection. Gummas (granulomatous lesions) may be widespread. Complications include dementia, meningitis, neuropathy, and thoracic aneurysm.

Diagnosis is by dark-field microscopy (primary or secondary) or serologic testing. The CDC provides treatment protocol for different populations. Treatment includes:

- **Primary, secondary, early tertiary:** penicillin G benzathine 104 million units IM in one dose
- **Tertiary:** penicillin G benzathine 2.4 million units IM weekly for 3 weeks

Posterior urethral valves

Posterior urethral valves is a urethral abnormality in males only where urethral valves have narrow slit-like openings that impede urinary flow and allow reverse flow, damaging urinary organs, which swell and become engorged with urine. Thirty percent will develop long-term kidney failure. Diagnosis is by fetal ultrasound, voiding cystourethrogram (VCUG) to evaluate extent of valvular abnormality and other urinary defects, endoscopy to examine inside of urinary tract/take tissue samples, blood tests to assess kidney function and electrolytes.

Symptoms	Treatment
Symptoms vary, depending upon severity: Small chest size with poor lung development and respiratory distress secondary to oligohydramnios (usually the most pressing clinical problem). Potter facies secondary to oligohydramnios. Limb deformities. Abdominal mass secondary to enlarged kidneys, bladder, or ascites. Sepsis, metabolic acidosis, and azotemia (increased blood levels of urea and other nitrogenous compounds) may develop.	Medical management: Supportive care, antibiotics, electrolytes, Foley catheter. Surgical management: Urinary diversion (usually closed after valve repair) and endoscopic ablation/resection to examine obstruction and remove valve leaflets.

Emergencies Unique to Neonates

Neonatal sepsis

Neonatal sepsis is a particular risk for preterm infants <1000 g and may be associated with a wide range of pathogens, both bacterial and viral. Early onset (≤72 hours) is usually related to maternal transmission and late onset (4 to 90 days) to invasive devices. Early onset sepsis most often is characterized by pneumonia and late onset by bacteremia and/or meningitis.

Symptoms	
Vary according to pathogen, onset, and primary site of infection: Nonspecific signs of respiratory distress, CNS irritation, and metabolic disorders. Pneumonia: tachypnea, sternal retraction, grunting respirations, cyanosis, and apneic periods. Meningitis: stupor, irritability, indications of increasing ICP, bulging anterior fontanel (but signs may be subtle in the neonate). Decreased cardiac output with pulmonary hypertension, signs of shock. Hypo- or hyperglycemia, metabolic acidosis. Jaundice. DIC. Necrotizing enterocolitis	
Laboratory findings (vary)	Treatment
Chest radiograph may show pneumonia. CT/MRI may show abscesses, obstructive hydrocephalus. Ultrasound may show abnormalities of ventricles and brain structures (meningitis). Thrombocytopenia <100,000 μL. WBC counts may not be elevated and may not show shift to left, especially initially. Immature to total neutrophil ratio increased. Clotting abnormalities (with DIC). Culture and sensitivities may not show infection because of small sample size. CSF: Elevated WBC count and protein level and positive culture (with meningitis). Increased C-reactive protein.	Intravenous antibiotics: Aminoglycoside and expanded-spectrum penicillin most common but vancomycin or oxacillin may be used for hospital-acquired infection. Surgical I &D of abscess. Ventriculoperitoneal shunt for hydronephrosis related to meningitis. NPO initially and then enteral feedings or TPN. Thermoregulation as indicated (radiant warmer, incubator). Maintenance of fluid balance and IV fluids as needed. Intubation/ventilation as needed.

Maternal STDs

Maternal **sexually transmitted diseases** can cause infection in the neonate. Common STDs include:

- **Chlamydia:** Infants most commonly exhibit conjunctivitis.
- **Gonorrhea:** Infants exposed to *Neisseria gonorrhoeae* during vaginal delivery most commonly develop bilateral conjunctivitis (ophthalmia neonatorum) if left untreated. In some cases, disseminated gonococcal infection (DGI) can occur in infants.
- **Syphilis (Congenital):** Infants may be asymptomatic, even with full system infection. Multiple system disorders and abnormalities can occur, including nonviral hepatitis with jaundice, hepatosplenomegaly, pseudoparalysis, pneumonitis, bone marrow failure, myocarditis, meningitis, anemia, edema associated with nephritic syndrome, and a rash on the palms of the hands and soles of the feet
- **Herpes:** Localized lesions may occur at 10–12 days. Disseminated infection may cause pneumonitis, hepatitis, and encephalitis.
- **HIV/AIDS:** Infants are asymptomatic at birth and may test falsely positive.
- **Trichomoniasis:** Infants may be born preterm and with low birth weight (<2500 g).

Necrotizing enterocolitis (NEC)

Necrotizing enterocolitis is an inflammatory bowel disease affecting primarily preterm/premature infants, characterized by an immature bowel that has suffered a hypoxic episode with resultant inflammation and necrosis of the intestinal wall, allowing gas into tissues of the wall, the portal venous system, and/or peritoneal cavity. It may result in infarction and/or perforation. The distal ileum and proximal colon are most commonly affected. The cause is not clearly understood, but appears related to an ischemic episode, colonization by bacteria, and excess/rapid enteral feedings. Mortality rates are about 30%.

Symptoms	Treatment
Gastric retention/ abdominal distention, vomiting (bilious). Periods of apnea. Occult or frank blood (25%) in stool. Pneumatosis intestinalis (gas in intestinal wall) (75%). Portal venous gas (10–30%). Decrease in urinary output. Jaundice. Unstable temperature.	Cessation of oral feeding and NG decompression. Systemic antibiotics. Correcting fluid and electrolyte imbalance. Surgical repair with bowel resection if necessary.

Complications include short gut syndrome, strictures, impaired nutrition, delayed growth, and cholestasis.

Neonatal fluid and electrolyte balance

Fluid and electrolyte balance must be maintained in the neonate. Fluid needs are usually estimated at 100 ml/kg but this may vary with changes in metabolic rate and output. Electrolytes that are of primary concern in neonates are calcium, sodium, and potassium.

	Normal value	Discussion
Ca	*Cord*: 8.2–11.2 mg/dL *0–10 days*: 17.6–10.4 mg/dL *11 days–2 years*: 9.0–11.0 mg/dL	Hypocalcemia: < 7 mg/dL is common with infants who are critically ill, IDM, suffered from asphyxia, or are preterm with very low birth weight.
Na	Neonate: 133–146 mEq/L	Hypernatremia: >150 mEq/L usually relates to dehydration, use of Na-containing solutions, congenital or acquired reduction in ADH, cerebral palsy, and intracranial hemorrhage. Hyponatremia: <130 mEq/L usually relates to overhydration, renal excretion from diuresis, or SIADH.
K	Neonate: 2.7–5.9 mEq/L	Hyperkalemia: >7 mEq/L may relate to renal failure, acidosis, or adrenal insufficiency. Hypokalemia: <3.5 mEq/L usually relates to excessive GI or renal fluid losses.

Neonatal electrolyte imbalances

Sodium (Na) regulates fluid volume, osmolality, acid-base balance, and activity in the muscles, nerves and myocardium. It is the primary cation (positive ion) in ECF, necessary to maintain ECF levels needed for tissue perfusion.
Normal neonatal value: 133–146 mEq/L
Hyponatremia: <133 mEq/L (Critical value <120)
Hypernatremia: >146 mEq/L (Critical value >160)

Hyponatremia develops in the neonate with excessive water gain or excessive sodium loss. Late symptoms include apnea, irritability, twitching, and seizures when serum sodium drops below 120 mEq/L, but infants are often asymptomatic. In the first days after birth, hyponatremia is usually secondary to excessive water gain (dilutional hyponatremia), reflected in a weight gain or absence of expected weight loss. Conditions causing dilutional hyponatremia include syndrome of inappropriate antidiuretic hormone (SIADH), renal dysfunction with decreased urine output, and overhydration. Treatment involves identifying and treating underlying cause, restricting fluid, and replacing sodium if necessary. Hypernatremia is caused by dehydration, excess use of sodium-containing solutions, and diabetes insipidus. Late symptoms include seizures. Underlying cause must be identified and treated.

Hypocalcemia: The ionized form of serum **calcium** is the only biologically available form in the body.

Cord: 8.2–11.2 mg/dL
0–10 days: 7.6–10.4 mg/dL
11 days to 1 yrs: 9.0–11.0 mg/dL
Critical value for hypocalcemia: <7 mg/dL
Signs of **hypocalcemia** in the neonate include jitteriness, irritability, stridor, tetany, high-pitched cry, seizures, and decreased myocardial contractility with decreased cardiac output. An electrocardiogram may show a prolonged QT interval and a flattened T wave. Early onset hypocalcemia usually presents in the first 3 days of life, and is associated with prematurity, birth asphyxia, and infants of diabetic mothers. Late onset hypocalcemia presents after the first week of life and is associated with DiGeorge syndrome, hyperphosphatemia, vitamin D deficiency, magnesium deficiency, diuretic therapy, and hypoparathyroidism. Hypocalcemia is treated with a slow infusion of calcium gluconate. Rapid infusion may cause bradycardia. Tissue infiltration with calcium causes necrosis, so administration site must be monitored.

Magnesium is the second most abundant intercellular cation.
Neonate: 1.5–2.2 mg/dL
Critical values: < 1.2 mg/dL and >3 mg/dL (neonates)
Hypermagnesemia most commonly results from maternal administration of magnesium prior to delivery. Maternal serum chemistries are reflected in newborn blood values. Magnesium is used in the pregnant woman as a tocolytic agent to stop preterm labor and also for treatment of pre-eclampsia. Signs of hypermagnesemia in an infant include hypotonia, hyporeflexia, constipation, low blood pressure, apnea, and marked flushing secondary to vasodilatation. Elevated magnesium blocks neurosynaptic transmission by interfering with the release of acetylcholine. Treatment is usually supportive, as the elevated serum magnesium will be cleared by the infant's kidneys. In severe cases, the infant may require respiratory and/or blood pressure support.

Hypomagnesemia in neonates occurs with preterm birth, respiratory distress syndrome, and neonatal hepatitis. Symptoms include:

- Neuromuscular excitability/ tetany
- Seizure and coma
- Tachycardia with ventricular arrhythmias
- Respiratory depression
- Treatment includes diagnosing underlying cause and magnesium replacement.

Serum potassium changes after birth

Electrolyte levels in the newborn reflect those of the mother at birth. Shortly after birth (within the first 24 to 72 hours) **serum potassium** concentrations are expected to rise without exogenous potassium delivery and with normal renal function, resulting from a shift of potassium from the intracellular space to the extracellular space. Potassium shift is more extreme in premature infants and can result in life-threatening hyperkalemia. Over the next several days, the potassium level will fall to normal in an infant with normally functioning kidneys. Preterm infants' serum electrolytes, including potassium, should be carefully monitored in the first 48 hours of life and until values have stabilized.
Normal neonatal values: 3.7 to 5.9 mEq/L

- Hyperkalemia: >6 mEq/L (Critical value: >6.5 mEq/L)
- Hypokalemia: <3.5 mEq/L (Critical value: <2.5 mEq/L)

Hyperkalemia

Neonatal hyperkalemia is a serum potassium level greater than 6 mEq/L in a non-hemolyzed blood sample. Squeezing the infant's heel too hard during blood collection can cause the sample to hemolyze and give an artificially elevated laboratory value. Cardiac manifestations of hyperkalemia include potentially fatal arrhythmias like bradycardia, tachycardia, supraventricular fibrillation, and ventricular fibrillation. EKG shows peaked T waves (earliest sign), and a widened QRS complex. Hyperkalemia must be treated promptly, especially if the blood potassium value is >7 mEq/L and the infant's electrocardiogram shows abnormalities. Treatment includes:

- Discontinue all potassium administration.
- Elevate the blood pH by inducing hyperventilation.
- Give sodium bicarbonate to shift extracellular potassium back inside cells.
- Administer insulin and/or inhaled albuterol to enhance the shift of extracellular potassium back inside cells. *Monitor glucose levels closely.*
- Increase excretion of potassium by giving furosemide (Lasix) or sodium polystyrene sulfonate (Kayexalate).
- Give calcium gluconate concurrently to help stabilize the myocardium and lessen the chance of the infant developing an arrhythmia.
- In extreme cases, consider dialysis or exchange transfusion.

Hyperbilirubinemia: Physiologic.

Hyperbilirubinemia, excess of bilirubin in the blood, is characterized by jaundice. Hyperbilirubinemia is evaluated according to the levels of direct (conjugated) bilirubin and/or indirect (unconjugated) bilirubin.
Direct/conjugated bilirubin levels increase with blockage of bile ducts, hepatitis or other liver damage, including drug reaction.
Indirect/unconjugated bilirubin levels increase with anemias (such as hemolytic disorders) and transfusion reactions.

Basic types of hyperbilirubinemia	
Physiologic	Common in newborns and usually benign, resulting from immature hepatic function and increased RBC hemolysis. Infants have larger red blood cells with a shorter life than adults, leading to more RBC destruction and resulting in an increased load of serum bilirubin, which the liver of the newborn cannot handle. Premature infants have an even greater physiologic jaundice as their RBCs live even shorter lives than the term infant's. Onset is usually within 24–48 hours, peaking in 72 hours for full term or 5 days for preterm infants and declining within a week. Phototherapy is the indicated treatment for total serum bilirubin ≥18 mg/dL

Hyperbilirubinemia: Hemolytic, breastfeeding associated, and breast milk jaundice

Basic types of hyperbilirubinemia (in addition to physiologic)	
Hemolytic	Caused by blood/antigen (Rh) incompatibility with onset in first 24 hours. Preventive treatment is RhoGAM® prenatally or postnatal exchange transfusion. This type of hyperbilirubinemia may also result from ABO incompatibility, but rarely requires treatment other than phototherapy.
Breastfeeding associated	Relates to inadequate calories during early breastfeeding with onset in 2–3 days. This slows the excretion of stool and allows bilirubin levels to rise. More frequent feeding with caloric supplements is usually sufficient, but phototherapy may be used for bilirubin 18–20 mg/dl.
Breast milk jaundice	May result from breast milk breaking down bilirubin and its being reabsorbed in the gut. Characterized by less frequent stools and onset in 4–5 days, peaking in 10–15

	days, but jaundice may persist for a number of weeks. Treatment involves discontinuing breastfeeding for 24 hours.

Hyperbilirubinemia: Indications for phototherapy and exchange transfusion

Phototherapy is often used to treat hyperbilirubinemia to prevent the need for exchange transfusion. For phototherapy, the infant is placed under special lights (15–20 cm above the infant) that will decrease the bilirubin levels in the blood. Indications include:

Weight	Serum bilirubin level
500–750 g	5–8 mg/dL
751–1000 g	6–10 mg/dL
1001–1250 g	8–10 mg/dL
1251–1500 g	10–12 mg dL

Exchange transfusions may be used for hyperbilirubinemia. Blood <72 hours old is used to maintain potassium levels. Indications include:

Weight	Serum bilirubin level
500–750 g	12–15 mg/dL
751–1000 g	>15 mg/dL
1001–1250 g	15–18 mg/dL
1251–1500 g	17–20 mg/dL

There are many risks associated with exchange transfusions, including vascular complications, such as emboli or thrombosis, often related to umbilical catheters. Cardiac complications include dysrhythmias and overload, leading to arrest. Clotting disorders may result from over-heparinization (reversed with protamine sulfate). Electrolyte and glucose abnormalities as well as infection may occur.

Hyperbilirubinemia: Phototherapy

Phototherapy is commonly used to treat hyperbilirubinemia and jaundice when the total serum bilirubin (TSB) indicates the infant is at risk. Phototherapy is a treatment in which the infant is placed under special lights that decrease the bilirubin levels in the blood. The lights usually consist of one tungsten halogen lamp or 4–8 white or blue fluorescent lights and a Plexiglas® shield. The infant is placed under these lights with a protective mask covering the eyes to prevent retinal toxicity. The lights should be 15–20 cm above the infant. The lights convert bilirubin into a water-soluble compound that can be excreted by the liver into bile and eventually into the infant's stool. The success of phototherapy is directly related to the quantity of body surface area that is exposed to the lights, so the infant is clad only in a diaper to expose the most skin to the light as possible.

Thermoregulation

At delivery, **minimize heat loss** while evaluating the newborn by following these steps:

- Dry the infant thoroughly (including hair) to minimize evaporative heat loss, and remove wet towels.
- Place a cap on the infant's head, as the head is the most significant area of heat loss.
- When the infant is to be weighed, cover the scales with a warm cloth to minimize conductive heat loss.
- Place infant in a warm environment such as:
- Skin-to-skin contact with mother, and cover them with a warm blanket.
- Bundled in warm blankets and given to mother to hold.

- Underneath a preheated warmer for further evaluation or resuscitation.
- Minimizing heat loss is especially important if the newborn is premature or has intrauterine growth restriction, but full term newborns also suffer hypothermia if they become chilled.

Cold stress/hypothermia in the neonate is a body temperature measurement of less than 36.5º C rectally with associated symptoms. Preterm neonates are especially vulnerable to cold stress, as they have limited ability to intrinsically create or conserve body heat. They do not shiver, have limited ability to constrict superficial blood vessels and have limited amounts of both subcutaneous and brown fat. Signs of cold stress include:

- Body is cool to touch, mottling of skin
- Central cyanosis and acrocyanosis
- Poor feeding, weak suck, increased gastric residuals, and abdominal distension
- Bradycardia
- Shallow respirations with tachypnea, apnea
- Restlessness and irritability
- Lethargy and decreased activity, weak cry
- Hypoglycemia
- Central nervous system depression with hypotonia
- Edema

There are a number of steps for **treatment of neonatal hypothermia**:

- Determine if the cause of hypothermia is from an abnormal physiological process in the infant or from environmental conditions.
- Do not rewarm the infant too rapidly because rapid rewarming may result in apnea or hypotension. Maintain the ambient temperature at 1 to 1.5°C higher than the infant's temperature. Oxygen consumption is not elevated when the difference between the skin temperatures and the environmental air temperature is less than 1.5°C.
- Increase the air temperature by approximately 1°C every hour until the infant's temperature is in the normal range and stable.
- Warm IV fluids with a blood-warming device prior to infusion to enhance warming.
- Closely monitor the infant's blood glucose levels, vital signs, and urinary output during rewarming.

Hyperthermia (rectal temperature greater than 37.0 ºC) can be caused by excessive heat from an external source (such as a radiant warmer set too high) or internally from a hypermetabolic state (such as a fever).

External heat source	Hypermetabolic
Core temperature < skin temperature. Skin warm and flushed	Core temperature > skin temperature. Skin cool to touch

Infants who are physiologically competent attempt to cool themselves when hyperthermia is caused by an external heat source by an extended posture, diaphoresis, and flushed, warm skin. Hyperthermia in the neonate can cause increased metabolic demands, vasodilatation, and increased fluid loss. An increased metabolic demand leads to an increased oxygen requirement, hypoxia, cyanosis, and breathing irregularities, such as tachypnea. Increased glucose consumption leads to hypoglycemia and its associated signs (jitteriness, lethargy, vomiting, or seizures). Peripheral vasodilatation helps cool the infant but may cause tachycardia and hypotension. Increased fluid losses contribute to tachycardia and hypotension. Signs of shock may develop with lethargy and decreased urine output. Dehydration may also cause electrolyte abnormalities.

Coarctation of the aorta

Coarctation of the aorta is a stricture of the aorta, proximal to the ductus arteriosus intersection. The increased blood pressure caused by the heart attempting to pump the blood past the stricture causes the heart to enlarge and increases blood pressure to the head and upper extremities while decreasing blood pressure and to the lower body and extremities. With severe stricture, symptoms may not occur until the ductus arteriosus closes, causing sudden loss of blood supply to the lower body.

Symptoms	Treatment
Difference in blood pressure between upper and lower extremities. Congestive heart failure symptoms in infants. Headaches, dizziness, and nosebleeds in older children. Increased risk of hypertension, ruptured aorta, aortic aneurysm, bacterial endocarditis, and brain attack.	Prostaglandin (alprostadil), such as Prostin VR Pediatric®, to reopen the ductus arteriosus for infants. Balloon angioplasty. Surgical resection and anastomosis or graft replacement (usually at 3–5 years of age unless condition is severe). Infants who have surgery may need later repair.

Pulmonic stenosis

Pulmonic stenosis is a stricture of the pulmonary artery that controls the flow of blood from the right ventricle to the lungs, resulting in right ventricular hypertrophy as the pressure increases in the right ventricle and decreased pulmonary blood flow. The condition may be asymptomatic or symptoms may not be evident until the child enters adulthood, depending upon the severity of the defect. Pulmonic stenosis may be associated with a number of other heart defects.

Symptoms	Treatment
Loud heart murmur. Congestive heart murmur. Mild cyanosis. Cardiomegaly. Angina. Dyspnea. Fainting. Increased risk of bacterial endocarditis.	Prostaglandin (alprostadil), such as Prostin VR Pediatric®, to reopen the ductus arteriosus for infants. Balloon valvuloplasty to separate the cusps of the valve for children. Surgical repair includes the (closed) transventricular valvotomy (Brock) procedure for infants and the cardiopulmonary bypass pulmonary valvotomy for older children.

Tetralogy of Fallot (TOF)

Tetralogy of Fallot (TOF) is a combination of 4 different defects:

- Ventricular septal defect (usually with a large opening)
- Pulmonic stenosis with decreased blood flow to lungs
- Overriding aorta (displacement to the right so that it appears to come from both ventricles, usually overriding the ventricular septal defect), resulting in mixing of oxygenated and deoxygenated blood
- Right ventricular hypertrophy
- Infants are often acutely cyanotic immediately after birth while others with less severe defects may have increasing cyanosis over the first year.

Symptoms	Treatment
Intolerance to feeding or crying, resulting in increased cyanotic "blue spells" or "tet spells" Failure to thrive with poor growth. Clubbing of fingers may occur over time. Intolerance to activity as child grows. Increased risk for emboli, brain attacks, brain abscess, seizures, fainting, or sudden death.	Prostaglandin (alprostadil), such as Prostin VR Pediatric®, to reopen the ductus arteriosus for infants. Total surgical repair at 1 year or younger is now the preferred treatment rather than palliative procedures formerly used.

Tricuspid atresia

Tricuspid atresia is lack of tricuspid valve between the right atrium and right ventricle so blood flows through the foramen ovale or an atrial defect to the left atrium and then through a ventricular wall defect from the left ventricle to the right ventricle and out to the lungs, causing oxygenated and deoxygenated bloods to mix. Pulmonic obstruction is common.

Symptoms	**Treatment**
Cyanosis obvious postnatally. Tachycardia and dyspnea. Increasing hypoxemia and clubbing in older children. Increased risk for bacterial endocarditis, brain abscess, and stroke.	Prostaglandin (alprostadil), to keep the ductus arteriosus and foramen ovale open if there are no septal defects. Numerous surgical procedures, including pulmonary artery banding, shunting from the aorta to the pulmonary arteries, Glenn procedure (connecting superior vena cava to pulmonary artery to allow deoxygenated blood to flow to the lungs), atrial septostomy to enlarge the opening between the atria, and the Fontan corrective procedure (usually done at 2–4 years after previous stabilizing procedures)

Hypoplastic left heart syndrome (HLHS)

Hypoplastic left heart syndrome (HLHS) is underdevelopment of the left ventricle and ascending aortic atresia causing inability of the heart to pump blood, so most blood flows from the left atrium through the foramen ovale to the right atrium and to the lungs with the descending aorta receiving blood through the ductus arteriosus. There may be valvular abnormalities as well. Mortality rates are 100% without surgical correction and 25% with correction.

Symptoms	**Treatment**
Symptoms may be mild until the ductus arteriosus closes at about 2 weeks causing a marked increase in cyanosis and decreased cardiac output: Increasing cyanosis. Decreased cardiac output leading to cardiovascular collapse	Prostaglandin (alprostadil), to keep the ductus arteriosus and foramen ovale open if there are no septal defects. Surgical procedures include a series of 3 staged operations: Norwood procedure connects the main pulmonary artery to the aorta, a shunt for pulmonary blood flow, and creates a large atrial septal defect. Glenn procedure. Fontan repair procedure. Heart transplantation in infancy is preferred in many cases, but the shortage of hearts limits this option.

Transposition of great arteries

Transposition of great arteries is the aorta and pulmonary artery arising from the wrong ventricle (aorta from the right ventricle and pulmonary artery from the left), so there is no connection between pulmonary and systemic circulation with deoxygenated blood being pumped back to the body and the oxygenated blood from the lungs is pumped back to the lungs. Septal defects may also occur, allowing some mixing of blood and the ductus arteriosus allows mixing until it closes. Symptoms vary depending upon whether mixing of blood occurs.

Symptoms	Treatment
Mild to severe cyanosis. Symptoms of congestive heart failure. Cardiomegaly develops in the weeks after birth. Heart sounds vary depending upon the severity of the defects.	Prostaglandin to keep the ductus arteriosus and foramen ovale open if there is no septal defect. Balloon atrial septostomy to increase size of foramen ovale, Surgical repair with cardiopulmonary bypass and aortic cross-clamping to transpose arteries to the normal position ("arterial switch") as well as repair septal defects and other abnormalities.

Ureteropelvic junction (UPJ) obstructions

Ureteropelvic junction (UPJ) obstruction is often discovered during prenatal ultrasounds, and is the most common cause of pediatric hydronephrosis (dilation of the renal pelvis). The most common cause of UPJ in the neonate is the lack of proper canalization of the renal pelvis during embryologic development. The obstruction can be mild or severe and may be asymptomatic in the newborn period. An abdominal mass may be the only sign of a UPJ obstruction with hydronephrosis in the newborn. The UPJ obstruction should be evaluated early with renal ultrasound, voiding cystourethrogram, and a renal scan to determine the degree of obstruction and the need for surgical correction. Another congenital anomaly occurs with UPJ obstruction in approximately 50% of cases, so both kidneys should be evaluated. If the obstruction is severe enough, surgical correction via renal pyeloplasty is performed to prevent renal damage.

Vesicoureteral reflux

Vesicoureteral reflux (VUR) is a condition in which urine from the bladder backflows into the ureters or kidneys. Normally, a valve exists at the junction of the ureters and the bladder, but in infants with VUR this valve is defective. Prenatally, VUR may be diagnosed by an ultrasound showing dilated ureters or renal pelvis. Postnatally, an infant with VUR may have an abdominal mass, or a urinary tract infection, or pyelonephritis. Nonspecific symptoms, such as respiratory distress, vomiting, failure to thrive, and renal failure may indicate pyelonephritis. VUR is more common in Caucasian children, and runs in families. It is more common in siblings who had VUR or if the parent has a history of VUR. Any infant with a history of a urinary tract infection or pyelonephritis should be evaluated for vesicoureteral reflux with a VCUG. Treatment includes waiting and watching (some children outgrow the condition), antibiotics to control urinary infections, and surgery (in severe cases).

Nutritional deficit

Maternal malnutrition can result in a profound **nutritional deficit** on the developing fetus and neonate. If malnutrition occurs during the stages of cell division, then cells may not divide properly, causing permanent damage. If malnutrition occurs when cells are enlarging, then correcting the nutritional deficit can reverse damage. Recommendations for maternal weight gain:

- Underweight: 28–40 lb
- Normal weight: 25–35 lb
- Overweight: 15–25 lb
- Obese: 15 lb

Malnourished or underweight mothers have increased perinatal losses and preterm births. Neonates often have lower Apgar score and low birth weight (<2500 g). Women with eating disorders are more likely to have infants that are small for gestational age. Vitamin and mineral deficiencies can cause abnormalities in the developing fetus.
Thiamine: Congestive heart failure, stillbirths
Folic acid: Megaloblastic anemia, neural tube defects
Vitamin D and calcium: Skeletal defects
Infants of obese and morbidly obese women are often macrosomic (large) and may suffer fetal distress, early neonatal death, meconium aspiration, shoulder dystocia, and/or complications from Caesarean birth.

Rapid assessment

The infant should be given a **rapid assessment** within seconds of birth to determine if the infant is at term, if the amniotic fluid is clear, if there is muscle tone, and if there are respirations or crying. If any of these conditions are not met, then the child should be placed under radiant heat and further resuscitation done. The basic steps to resuscitation include:

- Warming the infant after drying
- Positioning the infant and clearing the airway if necessary

- Stimulating and repositioning the infant
- The child should be evaluated throughout the initial procedures:
- Respirations: Rate and character of respirations should be noted as well as observation of chest wall movement.
- Heart rate: Should be >100 bpm, assessed with stethoscope or at the base of the umbilical cord.

APGAR delivery room assessment

Dr. Virginia Apgar developed the **APGAR** test in 1952. APGAR stands for **A**ppearance, **P**ulse, **G**rimace, **A**ctivity, and **R**espiration. The APGAR is the first test given to a newborn. It is used as a quick evaluation of a newborn's physical condition to determine if any emergency medical care is needed and is administered 1 minute and 5 minutes after birth. The test is administered more than once, as the baby's condition may change rapidly. It may be administered for a third time 10 minutes after birth if needed. The baby is rated on the five subscales and scores added together. A total score of ≥7 is a sign of good health.

Sign	**0**	**1**	**2**
Appearance (skin color)	Cyanotic or pallor over entire body	Normal, except for extremities	Entire body normal
Pulse (heart rate)	Absent	<100 bpm	>100 bpm
Grimace (reflex irritability)	Not responsive	Grimace	Infant sneezes, coughs, and recoils
Activity (muscle tone)	Absent	Flexed limbs	Infant moves freely
Respiration (breathing rate and effort)	Absent	Bradypnea, dyspnea	Good breathing and crying

Physical assessment

Head-Disproportionately large for body
Body-Long
Extremities-Short and in flexed position (feet usually dorsiflexed after breech birth)
Hands-Clenched
Neck-Short and chin resting on chest
Abdomen-Prominent
Hips-Narrow
Chest-Rounded
Weight-2500–4000 g (average about 3400) Physiologic weight loss is 5–10% for full term and 155 for preterm
Length-45–55 cm (average 50 cm)
Head circumference-32–38 cm (usually 2 cm greater than chest circumference)
Chest circumference-30–36 cm
Temperature-Temperature drops rapidly (skin temperature falls 0.3°C/minute) after birth with exposure to ambient room temperature but stabilizes within 8–12 hours. Temperature is usually measured by axillary method (for 3 minutes) and ranges from 36.3°C to 37.0°C.
Blood pressure-56–77/33–50 mm Hg
Pulse-140–120 bpm awake; 100 bpm asleep; 180 bmp crying
Respiration-30–60 per minute

Establishing airway

To **establish an airway**, the infant is placed supine with the head slightly extended in the "sniffing" position. A small neck roll may be placed under the shoulders to maintain this position in a very small premature infant. Once the proper position is established, the mouth and nose is suctioned (mouth first to prevent reflex inspiration of secretions when nose suctioned) with a bulb syringe or catheter if necessary. The infant's head can be turned momentarily to the side to allow secretions to pool in the cheek where they can be more easily suctioned and removed to establish the airway.

Stimulating the newborn is often all that is needed to initiate spontaneous respirations in the neonate. This tactile stimulation can be accomplished by gently rubbing the back or trunk of the infant. Another technique used to provide stimulation is flicking or rubbing the soles of the feet. Slapping neonates as stimulation is no longer practiced and should NOT be used.

ABCs of infant resuscitation

The **ABCs of infant resuscitation** are a device to help remember what order to do which steps of the resuscitation process. In this device, the letters stand for the following:

A—Airway	An airway should be established immediately; if there is no airway, air cannot be moved during resuscitation attempts. This step includes clearing the mouth and nose of secretions, and properly positioning the infant in the "sniff" position.
B—Breathing	This step involves initiating breathing after the airway has been established; this can be done with stimulation, supplemental oxygen, or through artificial ventilation.
C—Circulation	Once an airway and breathing have been established, then the circulation is considered; chest compressions may be indicated here or the administration of volume expanders and possibly epinephrine.

Resuscitation equipment

Minimum neonatal resuscitation equipment	
Temperature	Thermometer. Warmed drying towels, warmed swaddling blankets. Radiant warmer. Phototherapy equipment.
Respiration	Oxygen tank and hood, flow meter, humidifier, heater, tubing, nasal prongs. Bag and mask set-up (assorted sizes). Laryngoscope with size 0 and 1 blades. Endotracheal tubes, sizes 2.5–4. Bulb syringe, suction catheters sizes 6, 8, and 10 French, suction canister. Cardiorespiratory monitor, oxygen analyzer.
Fluids	IV needles and tubing, infusion pump, umbilical catheters (sizes 2.5 and 5 Fr). Blood pressure monitor, pulse oximeter. Isotonic saline, D10W. Sodium bicarbonate. If transfusions are done at this point, have a blood drainage system, volume expander, and blood warmer.
Drugs	Epinephrine. Naloxone.
Procedures	Various sterile surgical packs, dressings, chest tubes, scalpels, hemostat. Arterial blood gas equipment and portable x-ray machine.

Environmental

Heat stress

Children are particularly vulnerable to **heat-related illness**, especially when heat is combined with humidity, because of a low ratio of surface area to body mass and less capacity for perspiration. Heat-related illnesses occur when heat accumulation in the body outpaces dissipation, resulting in increased temperature and dehydration, which can then lead to thermoregulatory failure and multiple organ dysfunction syndromes. Each year in the United States, about 29 children die from heat stroke after being left in automobiles. At temperatures of 72–96°F, the temperature in a car rises 3.2° every 5 minutes, with 80% of rise within 30 minutes. Temperatures can reach 117°F even on cool days. There are 3 types of heat-related illness: Heat stress, heat exhaustion, and heat stroke.

Heat-related illness	
Heat stress	Increased temperature causes dehydration. Child may develop swelling of hands and feet, itching of skin, sunburn, heat syncope (pale moist skin, hypotension), heat cramps, and heat tetany (respiratory alkalosis). Treatment that is usually sufficient includes removing from heat, cooling, hydrating, and replacing sodium.

Heat exhaustion and heat stroke

Heat-related illness (In addition to heat stress)	
Heat exhaustion	Involves water or sodium depletion, with sodium depletion common in children and teenagers who are not acclimated to heat. Heat exhaustion can result in flu-like aching, nausea and vomiting, headaches, dizziness, and hypotension with cold clammy skin and diaphoresis. Temperature may be normal or elevated <106°. Treatment to cool the body and replace sodium and fluids must be prompt in order to prevent heat stroke. Careful monitoring is important and reactions may be delayed.
Heat stroke	Involves failure of the thermoregulatory system with temperatures that may be >106°F and can result in seizures, neurological damage, multiple organ failures and death. Exertional heat stroke often occurs in young athletes who engage in strenuous activities in high heat. Young children are susceptible to non-exertional heat stroke from exposure to high heat. Treatment includes evaporative cooling, rehydration, and supportive treatment according to organ involvement.

Hypothermia

Hypothermia occurs with exposure to low temperatures that cause the core body temperature to fall <95°F (35°C). Hypothermia may be associated with immersion in cold water, exposure to cold temperature, metabolic disorders (hypothyroidism, hypoglycemia, hypoadrenalism), or CNS abnormalities (head trauma, Wernicke disease). Many patients with hypothermia are intoxicated with alcohol or drugs. Diagnosis requires low-reading thermometers to verify temperature.

Symptoms	**Treatment**
Pallor, cold skin. Drowsiness, alterations in mental status, confusion. Severe shivering. Progression to shock, coma, dysrhythmias (T-wave inversion and prolongation of PR, QRS, and QT) including atrial fibrillation and AV block, and cardiac arrest.	Passive rewarming if cardiac status stable. Active rewarming (external) with immersion in warm water or heating blankets at 40°C, radiant heat. Active rewarming (internal) with warm humidified oxygen or air inhalation, heated IV fluids, and internal (bladder, peritoneal pleural, GI) lavage. Warming with extracorporeal circuit, such as arteriovenous or venovenous shunt that warms the blood. Supportive treatment as indicated.

Frostnip and frostbite

Frostnip is superficial reversible freeze injury. **Frostbite** is freezing damage to tissue, most often the nose, ears, and distal extremities. As frostbite develops, the affected part feels numb and aches or throbs, becoming hard and insensate as the tissue freezes, resulting in circulatory impairment, necrosis of tissue, and gangrene. There are 3 zones of injury:

- Coagulation (usually distal) is severe irreversible cellular damage.
- Hyperemia (usually proximal) is minimal cellular damage.
- Stasis (between other two zones) is severe but sometimes reversible.

Symptoms vary according to the degree of freezing:

- Partial freezing with erythema and mild edema, stinging, burning, throbbing pain.
- Full-thickness freezing with increased edema in 3–4 hours, edema, and clear blisters in 6–24 hours, desquamation with eschar formation, numbness and then aching and throbbing pain.
- Full-thickness and into sub-dermal tissue freezing with cyanosis, hemorrhagic blisters, skin necrosis and "wooden" feeling, severe burning, throbbing, and shooting pains.
- Freezing extends into subcutaneous tissue, including muscles, tendons, and bones with mottled appearance, non-blanching cyanosis and eventual deep black eschar.

Frostbite and freeze injuries

Prognosis is good with frostnip and fairly good for second-degree **freeze injuries** but poor for third- and fourth-degree freeze injuries. Determining the degree of injury can be difficult because some degree of thawing may have occurred prior to admission to the hospital. Treatment includes:

Initial warming	After warming
Rapid rewarming with warm water bath (40–42°C, 104–107.6°F) 10–30 minutes or until the frostbitten area is erythematous and pliable Treatment for generalized hypothermia	Debridement of clear blisters but not hemorrhagic blisters Aloe vera cream every 6 hours to blistered areas Dressings, separating digits Tetanus prophylaxis Ibuprofen 12 mg/kg daily in divided doses Antibiotic prophylaxis if indicated (Penicillin G 500,000 U IV every 6 hours for 24–72 hours

Coral snakes bites

About 45,000 **snakebites** occur in the United States each year, with about 8000 poisonous. In the United States, about 25 species of snakes are venomous. There are 2 types of snakes that can cause serious injury, classified according to the type of fangs and venom. **Coral snakes** have short, fixed, permanent fangs in the upper jaw and venom that is primarily neurotoxic, but may also have hemotoxic and cardiotoxic properties.

Signs and symptoms	Treatment
Wounds show no fang marks but there may be scratches or semi-circular markings from teeth. There may be little local reaction, but neurological symptoms may range from mild to acute respiratory and cardiovascular failure.	Cleanse wound thoroughly of dirt and debris and leave open or cover with dry dressing. Antibiotics not usually needed Administer antivenin immediately even without symptoms, which may be delayed. Tetanus toxoid or immune globulin

Pit viper bites

The second type of snake that can cause serious injury includes the **pit vipers**. Rattlesnakes, copperheads, and cottonmouths have erectile fangs that fold until they are aroused, and venom is primarily hemotoxic and cytotoxic but may have neurotoxic properties.

Signs and symptoms	Treatment
Wounds usually show 1–2 fang marks. Edema may begin immediately or may be delayed up to 6 hours. Pain may be severe. There may be a wide range of symptoms, including hypotension and coagulopathy with defibrination that can lead to excessive blood loss, depending upon the type and amount of venom. There may be local infection and necrosis.	Cleanse wound thoroughly and apply dressings as indicated. Tetanus toxoid or immune globulin. Analgesics, such as morphine sulfate Avoid NSAIDs and aspirin because of anticoagulation properties. Mark edema every 15 minutes. Antivenin therapy if indicated (observation for serum sickness if horse serum used). Prophylactic antibiotics for severe tissue necrosis. Platelets, plasma, or packed RBCs for coagulopathy.

Spider bites

Spider bites are frequently a misdiagnosis of a *Staphylococcus aureus* or MRSA infection, so unless the spider was observed, the wound should be cultured and antibiotics started. If the wound responds to the antibiotic, then it probably wasn't a spider bite. There are 2 main types of venomous spider bites:

- Producing neurological symptoms (Black widow)
- Producing local necrosis (brown recluse, yellow sac and hobos spiders)

Treatment includes:Cleanse wound and apply cool compress and elevate body part if possible.

Black widow bites	**Necrotic/ulcerated bites** (brown recluse, etc.)
Narcotic analgesics Nitroprusside to relieve hypertension Calcium gluconate 10% solution IV for abdominal cramps Latrodectus antivenin for those with severe reaction	There is no consensus on the best treatment as ulceration caused by the venom may be extensive and surgical repair with grafts may be needed. Treatment as for other necrotic ulcers, with moisture retentive dressings as indicated Hyperbaric oxygen therapy (HBOT) has been used in some cases of severe ulceration.

Human bites

Human "bites" occur when the teeth of one person injure another. This is not uncommon in contact sports. Intentional biting is common among children but usually presents mild injury. Human bites may also be the result of altercations and are referred to as "fist-bites." There are 3 common types of fist-bites:

- Closed fist bite resulting in small wound on the metacarpophalangeal joint of the middle finger. Bacteria enter the wound when the person extends the fingers, carrying bacteria to the extensor tendons, which can result in infection.
- Finger bite in which a finger may be partially or completely severed
- Puncture bite, usually on the face, from contact with another person's tooth

Immediate treatment of bites includes applying pressure to stop bleeding and then thoroughly flushing the wound with dilute Betadine®, dilute peroxide, or normal saline solution. Protective dressings should be applied. Large wounds or those with skin flaps or signs of more serious tissue injury may require surgical repair.

Animal bites

There is no one topical therapy for traumatic wounds because they vary so widely in the type and degree of injury. A scratch on the hand is treated very differently from a mauling that involves massive tissue injury or tissue loss. **Animal bites**, including human, are frequent causes of traumatic injury. Treatment includes:
Cleanse wound by flushing with 10–35cc syringe with 18-gauge angiocath (or size appropriate to wound) to remove debris and bacteria using normal saline or dilute Betadine® solution.
Hand, puncture, and infected wounds or those more than 12 hours old may be closed by secondary intention.
Moisture-retentive dressings as indicated by the size and extent of injury of wound left open. Dry dressings may be applied to injuries with closure by primary intention.
Topical antibiotics may be indicated although systemic antibiotics are commonly prescribed for animal bites.
Tetanus toxoid or immune globulin is routinely administered.

Insect stings

Insect stings: Honeybees, hornets, wasps, bumblebees, and yellow jackets	
Symptoms	**Treatment**
Honeybees have barbed stingers and can only sting once, but other bees have smooth stingers and can sting repeatedly. **Mild-local:** Pain, erythema, and swelling at bite site with small blister forming in about 4 hours and filling with milky dead tissue in 8 to 24 hours. **Moderate-Severe:** Swelling may extend to entire limb along with bruising for 12–48 hours. Area may be painful and itchy for several days. **Severe allergic/systemic:** Severe generalized edema, respiratory distress, nausea, vomiting, urticaria, faintness, and anaphylaxis syndrome.	**Mild-Moderate:** Remove stinger by scraping gently with sharp instrument. Wash with soap and water. Apply ice pack to reduce pain and swelling for 10–20 minutes at a time with 10–20 minutes between applications. Antihistamines. Topical corticosteroid for itching. Tetanus toxoid or tetanus immune globulin as indicated. **Severe allergic/systemic:** As for anaphylaxis, depending on degree of symptoms, including epinephrine.

Scorpion stings

Symptoms	Treatment
Note: Children <6 are most at risk of death from severe reactions. Symptoms vary widely depending on individual reaction and amount of venom. **Local** (most common): **Neurotoxic effects** include itching, redness, edema, and ascending hyperesthesia. Tap test: Paresthesia worsens if area tapped. **Cytotoxic effects** include development of macule or papule within an hour. Purpuric plaque becomes necrotic and ulcerates and venom spreads through the lymph system. **Nonlethal** response includes pain, induration, redness, and wheal. **Neurologic:** Severe wide-ranging symptoms include strokes, altered consciousness, muscle rigidity, paralysis, and seizures. **Multiple organ:** Can include hypertension, tachycardia, respiratory distress, generalized allergic response, dysphagia, hepatitis, priapism, acute tubular necrosis, DIC, hyperglycemia, lactic acidosis.	**Note:** Meperidine and morphine may potentiate symptoms. Hospital admission for 24 hours unless symptoms very mild. Cool compresses, acetaminophen, topical anesthetics for pain. Tetanus toxoid or tetanus immune globulin as needed. Antivenom (available only for Centruroides). Complex supportive care may include intubation and ventilation.

Fire ants bites

Insect bites: Fire ants	
Symptoms	**Treatment**
Note: Multiple bites, sometimes hundreds, are common. Deaths are rare but do occur if children have a severe systemic reaction or bites about the head and neck. **Local reaction:** A severely itching wheal develops and subsides in 30–60 minutes, followed by a blister within 4 hours. The blister fills with milky dead tissue in 8 to 24 hours with redness at base and severe itching and burning. The blister ruptures and crusts over within 72 hours but redness pain and itching may persist for days. **Systemic reaction:** Edema, urticaria, nausea, vomiting, bronchospasm, dyspnea, slurred speech, anaphylaxis.	**Local reaction:** Cold compresses, weak bleach solution (within 15 minutes of bites), or topical anesthetic for pain. Cleanse with soap and water without breaking blisters. NSAIDS for pain. Topical corticosteroids for itching. Antihistamines. Tetanus toxoid or tetanus immune globulin as needed. Systemic: As for anaphylaxis, depending on degree of symptoms, including epinephrine.

Toxic exposures

Children may be exposed to a wide range of **toxic exposures.** Contaminants can include toxins (produced by organisms) and toxicants (natural or synthetic chemicals). Contaminants are often produced by industry but may also be disseminated through acts of terrorism. Some types of exposure, such as from radiation, may have long-term effects not evident after initial exposure. Children tend to be more vulnerable to toxic exposures than adults. Risk factors for toxic exposures include:

- Parental employment with toxic substances
- Home built before1978 or with recent renovations
- Lack of adequate safety alarms for radon, carbon monoxide, and smoke
- Pica

Environmental toxic exposures can include pesticides, outdoor pollution (smoke, emissions), and indoor pollution (mold, lead, wood smoke, cigarette smoke). Children may develop toxic reactions from breastfeeding, skin contact, inhalation, or ingestion of contaminated food and fluids. Symptoms vary depending on the agent, but usually occur within 2 hours.

Carbon monoxide poisoning

Carbon monoxide (CO) poisoning occurs with inhalation of fossil fuel exhausts from engines, emission of gas or coal heaters, indoor use of charcoal, and smoke and fumes. The CO binds with hemoglobin, preventing oxygen carriage and impairing oxygen delivery to tissue. Diagnosis includes history, on-site oximetry reports, neurological examination, and CO neuropsychological screening battery (CONSB) done with patient breathing room air, CBC, electrolytes, ABGs, ECG, chest radiograph (for dyspnea).

Symptoms	Treatment
Cardiac: chest pain, palpitations, ↓ capillary refill, hypotension, cardiac arrest. CNS: malaise, nausea, vomiting, lethargy, stroke, coma, seizure. Secondary injuries: rhabdomyolysis with renal failure. Non-cardiogenic pulmonary edema. Multiple organs failure (MOF). DIC. Encephalopathy.	Immediate support of airway, breathing, and circulation. Non-barometric oxygen (100%) by non-breathing mask with reservoir or ETT if necessary. Mild: Continue oxygen for 4 hours with reassessment. Severe: hyperbaric oxygen therapy (usually 3 treatments) to improve oxygen delivery.

Cyanide poisoning

Cyanide poisoning, from hydrogen cyanide (HCN) or cyanide salts, can result from inhalation of burning plastics, intentional or accidental ingestion or dermal exposure, occupation exposure, ingestion of some plant products, manufacture of PCP, and sodium nitroprusside infusions. Inhalation of HCN causes immediate symptoms; ingestion of cyanide salts leads to symptoms within minutes. Diagnosis is by history, clinical examination, and normal PaO_2 and metabolic acidosis. Symptoms increase in severity and alter with the amount of exposure:

Symptoms	Treatment
Cardiovascular: tachycardia, hypertension, bradycardia, hypotension, and cardiac arrest. **Skin:** May appear pink or cherry-colored because of oxygen remaining in the blood. **CNS:** Headaches, lethargy, seizures, coma. **Respiratory:** Dyspnea, tachypnea, and respiratory arrest.	Supportive care as indicated. Removal of contaminated clothes. Gastric decontamination. Copious irrigation for topical exposure. **Antidotes**: Amyl nitrate ampule cracked and inhaled 30 seconds. Sodium nitrite (3%) 10 mL IV. Sodium thiosulfate (25%) 50 mL IV. (Children's doses of sodium nitrite and sodium thiosulfate adjusted according to hemoglobin level.)

Lead poisoning

Lead poisoning occurs with serum levels >10μg/dL although some children may experience cognitive impairment at lower levels. Lead poisoning is especially dangerous for developing children <7 because it interferes with normal cell function, especially in the nervous system, blood cells, and kidneys. Treatment involves removing source of lead and providing chelation therapy for levels >25 μg/dL. Agents used for chelation include calcium disodium ethylenediamine tetraacetate (CaNa2 EDTA), dimercaprol (BAL), d-penicillamine, or succimer (DMSA), usually for 5–7 days and then repeated.

- **Class I**-<9 μ/dL-Usually asymptomatic or slight neurological deficits.
- **Class II A**-10–14 μ/dL-Anemia. Mild cognitive, growth, and fine motor impairment.
- **Class II B**-15–19 μ/dL-Same as Class II A.

- **Class III**-20–44 µ/dL-Anemia. Fatigue, difficulty concentrating, headache. Motor impairment, tremors, paresis, paralysis. Abdominal pain, nausea, vomiting, constipation, weight loss.
- **Class IV**-45–69 µ/dL-Anorexia, vomiting, severe intermittent abdominal cramping. Hyperirritability. Increased lethargy. Blue-black lead line on gums.
- **Class V**->70 µ/dL-Encephalopathy, ataxia, seizures, coma, death.

Radiation sickness

Acute radiation sickness occurs with excess exposure to ionizing radiation. Symptoms vary according to the level of exposure, measured in gray (Gy) units. First symptoms can occur with entire body exposure to 1 Gy with >6 Gy often resulting in death. Those who survive have increased risk of cancer.

Gray	Initial	Delayed
1 to 2	Nausea and vomiting ≤6 hours	Increased weakness, lethargy, fatigue within 1 month
2 to 6	Nausea and vomiting in 2 hours, fever in 3, diarrhea in 8, and headache in 24	Increased weakness, lethargy, fatigue, hair loss, hematemesis, tarry stools, hypotension, and infections in 1 to 4 weeks
6 to 8	Nausea, vomiting, and fever in 1 hour, diarrhea in 3, and headache in 4	Symptoms as above occur within 1 week.
>8	Nausea and vomiting within 10 minutes and other symptoms (as above) within 1–2 hours	Symptoms as above occur immediately.

The severity of **acute radiation sickness** can be estimated based on details about a known exposure, onset of symptoms after exposure, blood tests that show WBC count depression or abnormal DAN, survey meter, and source of radiation. Treatment includes:

- Decontamination: Remove all clothes and wash or flush the skin with soap and water.
- Binding agents: With internal contamination by radioactive particles, treatment includes potassium iodide for radioactive iodine, Prussian blue for cesium and thallium, and diethylenetriamine pentaacetic acid (DTPA) for radioactive metals, such as plutonium.
- Bone marrow damage: Granulocyte colony-stimulating factor (filgrastim, pegfilgrastim) promotes leukocyte production to decrease risk of infections.

Supportive care: Medications may be given to control symptoms, such as nausea and vomiting and pain. If the child has received a lethal dose of radiation, comfort measures and hospice care should be provided.

Anthrax

Anthrax is caused by the biological agent *Bacillus anthracis*, which may be contracted from exposure to infected animals or through an act of terrorism. Treatment of choice for all types is ciprofloxacin 10 to 15 mg/kg every 12 hours (≤1 g/day for cutaneous). Standard precautions should be used. There are 3 primary types:

- **Cutaneous:** Blisters occur, ulcerating and forming necrotic lesions within 7 to 10 days. Infection is by direct contact with spores, such as from petting infected animals, and symptoms occur within 1 day. Use standard precautions.
- **Gastrointestinal:** Initially nausea, vomiting, loss of appetite, and fever and later acute abdomen within 1 to 7 days with ascites developing 2 to 4 days after initial symptoms and shock and/or death within 2 to 5 days.
- **Respiratory/Inhalation:** Non-specific respiratory symptoms, such as non-productive cough, malaise, diaphoresis, and myalgia usually occur in < 1 week but may be delayed for

≤2 months. Acute onset of severe respiratory distress occurs within 1 to 5 days of initial symptoms with shock/death in ≤36 hours.

Toxic ingestions

Treatment for **toxic ingestions** is related to the type of toxin and whether or not it is identified. Treatment includes:

- **Administering antidote** if substance is known and an antidote exists. Antidotes for common toxins include:
- Opiates: Naloxone (Narcan®)
- Toxic alcohols: Ethanol infusion and/or dialysis
- Acetaminophen: N-acetylcysteine
- Calcium channel blockers, beta-blockers: Calcium chloride, glucagon
- Tricyclic antidepressants: Sodium bicarbonate
- **GI decontamination** at one time was standard procedure (Ipecac® and gastric lavage followed by activated charcoal). It is no longer advised for routine use although selective gastric lavage may be appropriate if done within 1 hour of ingestion.
- **Activated charcoal** (1 g/kg wt) orally or per NG tube binds to many toxins if given within 1 hour of ingestion. It may also be used in multiple doses (q 4–6 hrs) to enhance elimination
- **Forced diuresis** with alkalinization of urine (>7.5) may prevent absorption of drugs that are weak bases or acids.

Acetaminophen toxicity

Acetaminophen toxicity from accidental or intentional overdose has high rates of morbidity and mortality unless promptly treated. Diagnosis is by history and acetaminophen level, which should be completed within 8 hours of ingestion if possible. Toxicity is plotted on the Rumack-Matthew nomogram with serum levels above 150 requiring antidote. Toxicity occurs with dosage >140 mg/kg in one dose or >7.5g in 24 hours. Symptoms occur in stages:

Symptoms	Treatment
Initial: Minor gastrointestinal upset. **Days 2–3**: Hepatotoxicity with RUQ pain and increased AST, ALT, and bilirubin. **Days 3–4**: Hepatic failure with metabolic acidosis, coagulopathy, renal failure, encephalopathy, nausea, vomiting, and possible death. **Days 5–12**: Recovery period for survivors.	GI decontamination with activated charcoal (orally or NG) within ≤4 hours. Gastric lavage if within 1 hour (may not be effective in small children because of size of NG tube). Antidote: 72-hour N-acetylcysteine (NAC) protocol includes 140 mg/kg initially and 70 mg/kg every 4 hours for 17 more doses (orally or IV). Children >40 kg IV administration of 150 mg/kg over 1 hour, diluted in 500 mL D5W% followed by maintenance dose of 100 mg/kg over 16 hours in 1000 mL D5W. Supportive therapy. (The antidote is most effective ≤8 hours of ingestion but decreases hepatotoxicity even >24 hours.)

Caustic ingestions

Caustic ingestions of acids (pH <7) such as sulfuric, acetic, hydrochloric, and hydrofluoric found in many cleaning agents and alkalis (pH >7) such as sodium hydroxide, potassium hydroxide, sodium tripolyphosphate (in detergents) and sodium hypochlorite (bleach) can result in severe injury and death. Acids cause coagulation necrosis in the esophagus and stomach and may result in metabolic acidosis, hemolysis, and renal failure if systemically absorbed. Alkali injuries cause liquefaction necrosis, resulting in deeper ulcerations, often of the esophagus, but may involve perforation and abdominal necrosis with multi-organ damage. Symptoms vary but include pain, dyspnea, oral burns, dysphonia, and vomiting. Diagnosis: detailed history, airway examination (oral intubation if possible), arterial blood gas, electrolytes, CBC, hepatic and coagulation tests, and radiograph, CT for perforations. Treatment includes:

- Supportive and symptomatic therapy
- NO ipecac, charcoal, neutralization, or dilution
- NG tube for acids only to aspirate residual
- Endoscopy in first few hours to evaluate injury/perforations
- Sodium bicarbonate for pH <7.10
- Prednisolone (alkali injuries)

Salicylate toxicity

Salicylate toxicity may be acute or chronic and is caused by ingestion of OTC drugs containing salicylates, such as ASA, Pepto-Bismol®, and products used in hot inhalers. Diagnosis is by ferric chloride or Ames test. Symptoms vary according to age and amount of ingestion, and co-ingestion of sedatives may alter symptoms.

Signs and symptoms	Treatment
<150 mg/kg: nausea and vomiting 150–300 mg/kg: Vomiting, hyperpnea, diaphoresis, tinnitus, and alterations in acid-base balance >300 mg/kg: Metabolic acidosis in children <4 but respiratory alkalosis and metabolic acidosis with alkalemia (pH >7.5) in older children. Chronic toxicity is more serious and includes hyperventilation, volume depletion, acidosis, hypokalemia, and CNS abnormalities.	Gastric decontamination with lavage (≤1 hour) and charcoal Volume replacement (D5W) Sodium bicarbonate 1–2mEq/kg Monitoring of salicylate concentration, acid-base, electrolytes every hour Whole-bowel irrigation (sustained release tablets)

Other Medical Emergencies

Sickle cell disease

Sickle cell disease is a recessive genetic disorder of chromosome 11, causing hemoglobin to be defective so that red blood cells (RBCs) are sickle-shaped and inflexible, resulting in their accumulating in small vessels and causing painful blockage. While normal RBCs survive 120 days, sickled cells may survive only 10–20 days, stressing the bone marrow that can't produce fast enough and resulting in anemia. Different types of **crises** occur (aplastic, hemolytic, vaso-occlusive, and sequestrating), which cause infarctions in organs, severe pain, damage to organs, and rapid enlargement of liver and spleen. Sickle cell disease and crisis treatment includes:

- Intravenous fluids to prevent dehydration
- Analgesics (morphine) during painful crises
- Folic acid for anemia
- Oxygen for congestive heart failure or pulmonary disease
- Blood transfusions with chelation therapy to remove excess iron OR erythropheresis, in which red cells are removed and replaced with healthy cells, either autologous or from a donor
- Hematopoietic stem cells transplantation is the only curative treatment.

Hemophilia

Hemophilia is an inherited disorder in which the child lacks adequate clotting factors. There are 3 types:

- Type A: lack of clotting factor VII (90% of cases)
- Type B: lack of clotting factor IX
- Type C: Lack of clotting factor XI (affects both sexes, rarely occurs in the US)

Both Type A and B are usually X-linked disorders, affecting only males. The severity of the disease depends on the amount of clotting factor in the blood. Babies often show symptoms when more active, crawling or walking, with frequent bruises.

Symptoms	Treatment
Bleeding with severe trauma or stress (mild cases) Unexplained bruises, bleeding, swelling, joint pain Spontaneous hemorrhage (severe cases), often in the joints but can be anywhere in the body Epistaxis	Desmopressin parenterally or nasally to stimulate production of clotting factor (mild cases) Infusions of clotting factor from donated blood or recombinant clotting factors (genetically-engineered) Infusions of plasma (Type C)

Disseminated intravascular coagulation (DIC)

Disseminated intravascular coagulation (DIC) (consumption coagulopathy) is a secondary disorder that is triggered by another, such as trauma, congenital heart disease, necrotizing enterocolitis, sepsis, and severe viral infections. DIC triggers both coagulation and hemorrhage through a complex series of events that includes trauma that causes tissue factor (transmembrane glycoprotein) to enter the circulation and bind with coagulation factors, triggering the coagulation cascade. This stimulates thrombin to convert fibrinogen to fibrin, causing aggregation and destruction of platelets and forming clots that can be disseminated throughout the intravascular system. These clots increase in size as platelets adhere to the clots, causing blockage of both the microvascular systems and larger vessels, and this can result in ischemia and necrosis. Clot formation triggers fibrinolysis and plasmin to breakdown fibrin and fibrinogen, causing destruction of clotting factors, resulting in hemorrhage. Both processes, clotting and hemorrhage continue at the same time placing the patient at high risk for death, even with treatment.

The onset of **symptoms of DIC** may be very rapid a slower chronic progression from a disease, such as in children with large vascular malformations.

Symptoms	Treatment (varies)
Bleeding from surgical or venous puncture sites Bleeding from umbilicus and trachea in newborns Evidence of GI bleeding with distention, bloody diarrhea Hypotension and acute symptoms of shock Petechiae and purpura with extensive bleeding into the tissues Laboratory abnormalities: Prolonged prothrombin and partial thromboplastin times Decreased platelet counts and fragmented RBCs Decreased fibrinogen	Identifying and treating underlying cause Replacement blood products, such as platelets and fresh frozen plasma Anticoagulation therapy (heparin) to increase clotting time Cryoprecipitate to increase fibrinogen levels Coagulation inhibitors and coagulation factors

Idiopathic thrombocytopenic purpura (ITP)

The autoimmune disorder **idiopathic thrombocytopenic purpura (ITP)** causes an immune response to platelets, resulting in decreased platelet counts. It may be triggered by viral infections.

The acute form is usually short lasting and affects children, who often go into remission in 6–12 months. The chronic form affects primarily adults but also children (about 5%). Platelet counts after the first week of life are about the same in children as adults, 150,000–400,000 per cu/ml. With ITP, they may be as low as 0 or 100,000 in less severe cases. A count of about 30,000 is necessary to prevent intracranial hemorrhage, the primary concern. ITP is usually not life threatening and can be controlled.

Symptoms	Treatment
Bruising and petechiae with hematoma in some cases Epistaxis Increased menstrual flow in females, post-puberty	Corticosteroids depress immune response and increase platelet count. Splenectomy may be indicated for chronic conditions. Platelet transfusions Avoid aspirin or ibuprofen

Neutropenia and fever

Neutropenia occurs with a decrease in absolute neutrophil count (ANC), putting the child at risk for severe sepsis and death. Neutropenia may occur because of decreased neutrophil destruction or production. Causes include leukemia, aplastic anemia, vitamin B12 deficiency, autoimmune disorders, chemotherapeutic agents, and congenital neutropenia.
Normal values include:

- 1 year: 1500–8500.
- 10 years: 1800–8000.
- 18 years: 1800–7700.

Risk of infection increases markedly when the ANC falls to 1000 and is severe at 500. Symptoms may be nonspecific or absent, so neutropenia may be undiagnosed before infection occurs. Any child with neutropenia and fever should be hospitalized for probable infection and treated with broad-spectrum antibiotics. Super infections, especially fungal, are common. Precautions include shielding from those with infections, private room with ANC <1000, and prohibiting fresh flowers, fresh salads, and unpeeled fruits and vegetables. Good hygiene is critical, and the perineal area should be washed after every BM, especially with infants.

Tumor lysis syndrome

Tumor lysis syndrome is a severe reaction to cancer treatment, usually for large tumors or cancers that proliferate rapidly but respond to treatment, including leukemia and non-Hodgkin's lymphoma. As large numbers of tumor cells die, a toxic reaction occurs that can result in acute renal failure, hyperuricemia, and electrolyte imbalances, including increased levels of potassium and phosphate and decreased calcium. Some children exhibit symptoms prior to treatment, putting them at especially high risk. Symptoms can include nausea, vomiting, hypervolemia, heart failure, dysrhythmias, tetany, and muscle cramping. Sudden death may occur, usually ≤ 72 hours of initiating cytotoxic chemotherapy. Careful monitoring is essential to providing preventive measures, including 3 times daily laboratory monitoring of renal status and electrolytes during the first 72 hours of therapy. Fluid status must be monitored and IV fluids provided. Treatments include allopurinol or rasburicase for hyperuricemia, isotonic sodium bicarbonate to keep urine alkaline, diuretics for fluid overload, electrolyte control, and hemodialysis.

Adrenocortical insufficiency (Addison's disease)

Adrenocortical insufficiency (Addison's disease) is caused by damage to the adrenal cortex, related to a variety of causes, such as autoimmune disease or genetic disorders, but most cases in children relate to destructive lesions or neoplasms. Without treatment, the condition is life threatening. Symptoms may be vague and the condition undiagnosed until 80–90% of the adrenal cortex has been destroyed.

Signs and symptoms	Treatment
Chronic weakness and fatigue Abdominal distress with nausea and vomiting Salt or licorice craving, resulting from deficiency of aldosterone Pigmentary changes in skin and mucous membranes, hyperpigmentation Hypotension and small heart size Hypoglycemia Recurrent seizures (common in children)	Hormone replacement therapy with glucocorticoids (cortisol) and mineralocorticoids (aldosterone) may be taken orally or monthly parenteral injections or subcutaneous implantation of desoxycorticosterone acetate every 9–12 months. During times of stress or illness, the demand for glucocorticoids may increase and dosages up to 3 times the normal dosage may be needed to prevent an acute crisis.

Acute adrenal insufficiency (adrenal crisis)

Acute adrenal insufficiency (adrenal crisis) is a sudden, life-threatening condition resulting from an exacerbation of primary chronic adrenal insufficiency (Addison's disease), often precipitated by sepsis, surgical stress, adrenal hemorrhage related to septicemia, anticoagulation complications, and cortisone withdrawal related to decreased dose or inadequate dose to compensate for stress. Acute adrenal insufficiency may occur in those who do not have Addison's disease, such as those who have received cortisone for various reasons, usually a minimum of 20 mg daily for at least 5 days.

Signs and symptoms	Treatment (Immediate)
Fever Nausea and vomiting, abdominal pain, dehydration Weakness and general fatigue Disorientation, confusion Hypotensive shock Electrolyte imbalance with hyperkalemia, hypercalcemia, hypoglycemia and hyponatremia	IV fluids in large volume Glucocorticoids 50% dextrose if indicated (hypoglycemia) Mineralocorticoids may be needed after intravenous solutions. The precipitating cause must be identified and treated as well.

Cushing syndrome

Cushing syndrome is caused by increased production of cortisol from a variety of etiologies.

- Excess of ACTH causing adrenal hyperplasia
- Hypersecretion of glucocorticoids usually related to neoplasms
- Extra-pituitary neoplasms causing autonomous secretion of ACTH
- Iatrogenic, resulting from exogenous corticosteroids (the most common cause in children)

Signs and symptoms	**Treatment**
Changes in fat distribution with truncal obesity, supraclavicular fat pads, and fat pads on back of neck, moon face, large abdomen Weight gain Increased bruising and poor wound healing Hypertension Hypokalemia Hyperglycemia Virilization with increased hirsutism and acne Kyphosis with depressed linear growth	Treatment depends upon the cause. If caused by medications, such as prednisone, slow withdrawal of the medication should reverse symptoms over time. Giving medications in early morning on alternate days may reduce symptoms. In some cases, bilateral adrenalectomy and replacement hormone therapy (as for Addison's disease) is indicated.

Diabetes mellitus

Diabetes mellitus is the most common metabolic disorder in children, affecting about 1.5 million children and adolescents with 70–85% having type 1 and the rest having type 2. The peak age of onset for both types is 10–12 in girls and 12–14 in boys:

Type 1 (Insulin dependent)	Type 2 (Insulin resistant)
Immune-mediated form with insufficient insulin production because of destruction of pancreatic beta cells. **Symptoms** include: Pronounced polyuria and polydipsia. Short onset. May be overweight, or recent weight loss. Ketoacidosis present on diagnosis. **Treatment**: Insulin as needed to control blood sugars. Glucose monitoring 1–4 times daily. Diet control with carbohydrate control. Exercise.	Insulin resistant form with defect in insulin secretion. **Symptoms** include: Long onset. Obese with no weight loss or significant weight loss. Mild or absent polyuria and polydipsia. May have ketoacidosis or glycosuria without ketonuria. Androgen-mediated problems such as hirsutism and acne. Hypertension. **Treatment**: Diet, exercise, and oral medications. Glucose monitoring.

Target plasma glucose and A1C levels for type 1 diabetes

American Diabetes Association Clinical Practice Recommendations for **target plasma glucose and A1C levels** for type 1 diabetes in infants and youths varies according to age.

Age	Plasma glucose before meals	Plasma glucose HS (night)	A1C	Discussion
0–6	100–180 mg/dL	110–200	>7.5% and <8.5%	Increased risk for hypoglycemia
6–12	90–180	100–180	<8%	Risks for hypoglycemia remain high and complications are usually low pre-puberty.
13–19	90–130	90–150	<7.5%	Individualized goals may be lower, based on benefits and risks.

Hypoglycemia can result in permanent cognitive impairment in children <5, so management must recognize that normal plasma glucose levels are usually not attainable. Adolescents often have A1C about 1% higher than adults although the increased use of insulin pumps has helped patients maintain proper levels.

Ketoacidosis

Ketoacidosis is a complication of diabetes mellitus. Inadequate production of insulin results in glucose being unavailable for metabolism, so lipolysis (breakdown of fat) produces free fatty acids (FFAs) as an alternate fuel source. Glycerol in both fat cells and the liver is converted to ketone bodies (β-hydroxybutyric acid, acetoacetic acid, and acetone), which are used for cellular metabolism less efficiently than glucose. Excess ketone bodies are excreted in the urine (ketonuria) or exhalations. The ketone bodies lower serum pH, leading to ketoacidosis.

Signs and symptoms	Treatment
Kussmaul respirations: hyperventilation to eliminate buildup of carbon dioxide, associated with "ketone breath" Fluid imbalance, including loss of potassium and other electrolytes from cellular death, resulting in dehydration and diuresis with excess thirst. Cardiac arrhythmias, related to potassium loss, can lead to cardiac arrest. Hyperglycemia, with glucose levels above normal. **Normal glucose values**: Neonate: 40–60 mg/dL. <12 months: 50–90 mg/dL. >12 months: 60–100 mg/dL	Insulin therapy by continuous infusion initially. Rehydration and electrolyte replacement. Glucose monitoring. Ketone monitoring.

Acute hypoglycemia/insulin reaction

Acute hypoglycemia (insulin reaction) can cause damage to the central nervous and cardiopulmonary systems, interfering with development of the brain and causing neurological impairment. The most common cause is excess insulin dosage for needs. This may occur as a result of improper dosing, inadequate dietary intake, strenuous exercise, or vomiting. Prompt treatment is essential to avoid coma and death.

Signs and symptoms	Treatment
Blood glucose <50 mg/dL Central nervous system: seizures, altered consciousness, lethargy, and poor feeding with vomiting, myoclonus, respiratory distress, diaphoresis, hypothermia, and cyanosis	Oral sugar in the form of a liquid, juice, or candy may be given if the child is alert and response. IV glucose/glucagon administration to elevate blood glucose levels

Metabolic and respiratory acidosis

Factors	Metabolic	Respiratory
Patho-physiology	Increase in fixed acid and inability to excrete acid or loss of base, with compensatory increase of CO_2 excretion by lungs	Hypoventilation and CO_2 retention, with renal compensatory retention of bicarbonate (HCO_3) and increased excretion of hydrogen
Laboratory	Decreased serum pH and PCO_2 normal if uncompensated, and decreased if compensated; Decreased HCO_3; Urine pH <6 if compensated	Increased serum pH and increased PCO_2;Increased HCO_3 if compensated and normal if uncompensated;Urine pH >6 if compensated
Causes	DKA, lactic acidosis, diarrhea, starvation, renal failure, shock, renal tubular acidosis, starvation	COPD, overdose of sedative or barbiturate, obesity, severe pneumonia atelectasis, muscle weakness (Guillain-Barré), mechanical hypoventilation
Symptoms	Neuro/muscular: drowsiness, confusion headache, coma. Cardiac: Decreased BP, arrhythmias, flushed skin. GI: nausea, vomiting, abdominal pain, diarrhea. Respiratory: Deep inspired tachypnea	Neuro/muscular: drowsiness, dizziness, headache, coma, disorientation, seizures. Cardiac: Flushed skin, VF, decreased BP. GI: absent. Respiratory: Hypoventilation with hypoxia.

Metabolic and respiratory alkalosis comparison

Factors	Metabolic	Respiratory
Patho-physiology	Decreased strong acid or increased base, with compensatory CO_2 retention by lungs	Hyperventilation and increased excretion of CO_2, with compensatory HCO_3 excretion by kidneys
Laboratory	Increased serum pH; PCO_2 normal if uncompensated and increased if compensated; Increased HCO_3; Urine pH >6 if compensated	Increased serum pH; Decreased PCO_2; HCO_3 normal if uncompensated and decreased if compensated; Urine pH >6 if compensated
Causes	Excessive vomiting, gastric suctioning, diuretics, potassium deficit, excessive mineralocorticoids and $NaHCO_3$ intake	Hyperventilation associated with hypoxia, pulmonary embolus, exercise, anxiety, pain, and fever; Encephal-opathy, septicemia, brain injury, salicylate overdose, mechanical hyperventilation
Symptoms	Neuro/muscular: dizziness, confusion, nervousness, anxiety, tremors, muscle cramping, tetany, tingling, seizures. Cardiac: Tachycardia and arrhythmias. GI: Nausea, vomiting, anorexia. Respiratory: Compensatory hypoventilation.	Neuro/muscular: Light-headed, confused, lethargic. Cardiac: Tachycardia and arrhythmias. GI: Epigastric pain, nausea and vomiting. Respiratory: Hyperventilation

Cystic fibrosis

Cystic fibrosis (mucoviscidosis) is a progressive congenital disease that particularly affects the pancreas and lungs causing digestive and respiratory problems. It is caused by a genetic defect that affects sodium chloride movement in cells, including mucosal cells that line the lungs, causing the production of thick mucus that clogs the lungs and provides a rich medium for bacteria. While most patients with cystic fibrosis at one time died in childhood, the life expectancy is now about 37 years. Cystic fibrosis patients usually suffer from recurrent respiratory infections of the lower respiratory tract. The most common infective agents are *Pseudomonas aeruginosa* and *Burkholderia cepacia* complex. Patients with chronic infections serve as reservoirs for patient-to-patient transmission of infection, with proximity and duration of contact as precipitating factors. Cystic fibrosis patients should be maintained on universal and droplet precautions and, when hospitalized, placed in private rooms or cohorted with someone with the same pathogen.

Marfan syndrome

Marfan syndrome is a genetic disorder of the connective tissue related to protein metabolism. Connective tissue, such as tendons, ligaments, heart valves, and blood vessels are often defective and weak, and the child is at risk for aortic dissection. Depending upon the severity, children may be restricted from strenuous activities, such as team sports, especially contact sports that may result in chest trauma, or isometric exercises, such as weight lifting.

Traits	Treatment
Tall, thin stature with loose joints, with the long bones disproportionately long. Scoliosis, flat feet. Pectus carinatum (pigeon chest) or pectus excavatum (funnel chest). Long, narrow face with high arched roof of mouth and crowding of teeth. Dislocation of lenses of eyes and sometimes retinal detachment, myopia. Aortic dilatation (with risk of dissection), cardiac valve disorders with heart murmur. Stretch marks. Abdominal/inguinal hernia. Sleep apnea (rare).	Prophylactic antibiotics to prevent endocarditis. β-Blockers if aorta dilated to delay expansion. Prophylactic surgery to repair aortic dilation. Surgical repair of dissecting aortic aneurysm.

Contact dermatitis

Contact dermatitis is a localized response to contact with an allergen, resulting in a rash that may blister and itch. Common allergens include poison oak, poison ivy, latex, benzocaine, nickel, and preservatives, but there is a wide range of items, preparations, and products to which children may react.

Treatment includes:

- Identifying the causative agent through evaluating the area of the body affected, careful history, or skin patch testing to determine allergic responses
- Corticosteroids to control inflammation and itching, usually topical
- Soothing oatmeal baths
- Caladryl® lotion to relieve itching
- Antihistamines to reduce allergic response
- Gentle cleansing of lesions and observation for signs of secondary infection
- Antibiotics only for secondary infections as indicated
- Rash usually left open to dry
- Avoidance of allergen to prevent recurrence

Folliculitis and impetigo

Folliculitis is bacterial infection of the hair follicles, often on the face, resulting in pustules, erythema, and crusts that are painful and itchy. Recently, there has been an increase in cases of community-acquired methicillin-resistant *Staphylococcus aureus* (MRSA) folliculitis infections. Folliculitis may occur as a primary or secondary infection and may result from chronic nasal colonization of MRSA.
Treatment includes:

- Antibacterial soaps
- Topical (Bactroban®) and oral antibiotics
- **Impetigo** is a contagious itchy bacterial infection of the skin, commonly on the face or hands, causing clusters of blisters or sores, especially in children. Group A streptococcus usually causes small blisters that crust over. *Staphylococcus aureus* usually causes larger blisters that may be bullous and cause lesions 2–8 cm in size that persist for months. Treatment includes:
- Avoid scratching.
- Gently cleanse area with soap and water.
- Apply topical Bactroban® 3 times daily until healed.

Erysipelas

Erysipelas is a superficial bacterial infection, primarily of the face or legs, involving the cutaneous lymphatic system and invading the skin in areas of trauma. Facial erysipelas is usually caused by group A streptococcus following a nasopharyngeal infection. Infections on the legs are more often related to non-group A streptococcus. The infection spreads rapidly with streaking and clearly demarcated erythema and cellulitis. Local lymph nodes become inflamed, sometimes resulting in lymphedema because of damage to lymph nodes. Erysipelas most commonly affects children and the elderly. Treatment includes:

- Bed rest with elevation of affected limb and warm saline packs to improve circulation
- Oral antibiotic (usually penicillin G and penicillin VK); IV antibiotics may be indicated for severe cases
- Hospitalization is recommended for severe cases or those who are very young, elderly, or immunocompromised.
- Analgesics to control pain

Staphylococcal scalded skin syndrome (SSSS)

Staphylococcal scalded skin syndrome (SSSS) is a superficial partial-thickness infection of the skin caused by toxins produced by a localized *Staphylococcus aureus* infection, resulting in generalized erythema followed in 24–48 hours with blisters that rupture and peel off, leaving large areas of superficial necrosis and denuded skin, giving the skin a burned or "scalded" appearance. It is most common in neonates and children under 5. Pain is usually mild unless the infection is very widespread. Treatment includes:

- IV antibiotics (such as flucloxacillin) are usually needed initially, followed by a course of oral antibiotics.
- Maintenance of fluids and electrolytes
- Debridement of skin
- Moisture-retentive dressings, such as foam dressings, sheet hydrogels, and alginates, avoiding adhesives

- Excessive tissue loss may be treated the same as partial-thickness burns.

Necrotizing fasciitis

Necrotizing fasciitis is a rapidly spreading infection of the soft tissues involving extensive necrosis of the fascia and subcutaneous tissue as well as destruction of the vasculature with thrombosis. It most often occurs in the extremities after a minor infection. The most common organisms are group A β-hemolytic streptococci but there may be polymicrobial infections or other causative agents. It may result from surgical procedures, including cardiac catheterization. The infection begins with pain, edema, fever, toxemia, and cellulitis that spread rapidly, becoming increasingly cyanotic as tissue and perfusion is impaired. Bullae form and progress to necrosis and gangrene and sepsis within 3–5 days. Mortality rates are 25%. Treatment includes:

- Aggressive extensive surgical debridement of all non-viable tissue. Repeat surgical debridement may be necessary.
- Antibiotic therapy
- Wound care as indicated by the extent of the wound with careful monitoring to determine if wound is deteriorating
- IV immunoglobulin may be used.

Hyphema

Hyphema is the accumulation of hemorrhaging blood in the anterior chamber of the eye after an injury. It is usually caused by a projectile hitting the eye and resulting in blunt or penetrating trauma. Hyphema is classified according to degree.
Grade 1: blood (layered) occupies <1/3 of chamber.
Grade 2: blood (filling) occupies 1/3–1/2 of chamber.
Grade 3: blood (layered) occupies >1/2 of chamber.
Grade 4: clotted blood occupies total chamber.

Signs and symptoms	Treatments
Increased intraocular pressure >22 mm Hg initially (in about 1/3 of patients) followed by reduction in 2–6 days for those with less than 3/4 filling of chamber. Those with >3/4 filling of chamber may have continued increase in intraocular pressure. Secondary hemorrhage may occur, especially in children and African Americans.	Patch and shield for injured eye. Tylenol for analgesia (NSAIDs should be avoided). Topical steroids. Systemic aminocaproic acid to prevent secondary hemorrhage. Anti-glaucoma topical medications, such as Alphagan®, for increased IOP.

Conjunctivitis

Conjunctivitis is a common eye disorder that may be due to various causes, including bacterial, viral, systemic disease, or allergy.

- **Bacterial conjunctivitis** may be secondary to *Staphylococcus* and *Streptococcus* (most common) but can be from many organisms, including *Gonococcus* and *Chlamydia*. All bacterial cases produce purulent discharge and may be treated with topical drops, but gonococcal disease may deteriorate rapidly, requiring IV ceftriaxone. Chlamydial disease is treated with tetracycline or erythromycin.
- **Viral conjunctivitis** is commonly due to adenovirus and is associated with a syndrome, including pharyngitis and fever. Discharge is watery, and disease is usually self-limited. Topical antibiotics may limit secondary infection but are not usually advised.
- **Systemic disease**, such as Sjögren's syndrome, and **foreign bodies**, may lead to conjunctivitis. Treatment is usually artificial tears.

- **Allergic conjunctivitis** is often associated with other atopic diseases, and antihistamines and topical steroids may be of use.

Retinal detachment

Retinal detachment occurs when the retinal pigment epithelial (RPE) layer separates from the underlying sensory layer. Retinal detachment may occur as the result of traumatic injury, systemic disease (such as diabetes), or ocular malformation. Diagnosis includes checking visual acuity and examining dilated fundus with indirect ophthalmoscope and Goldman 3-mirror to create a detailed retinal diagram. **Symptoms** include: Painless visual changes, such as floaters, "cobwebs," photopsia (flashes of light), shadow over vision, or loss of central vision. **Treatment**: Surgical repair (pneumatic retinopexy, scleral buckling, or vitrectomy)

Types of retinal detachment	
Rhegmatogenous	A tear occurs in the sensory retina and liquid vitreous seeps through, detaching the RPE.
Traction	Bands of scar tissue provide traction that pulls on retina, usually related to diabetes, vitreous hemorrhage, or retinopathy of prematurity.
Exudative	The choroid produces serous fluid under the retina, usually related to uveitis or macular degeneration.
Combination	Combinations of other types with varying presentation

Corneal abrasions

Corneal abrasion results from direct scratching or scraping trauma to the eye, often involving contact lenses, causing a defect in the epithelium of the cornea. Infection with corneal ulceration can occur with abrasions. Determining the cause and source of the abrasion is important for treatment as organic sources pose the danger of fungal infection and soft contact lenses pose the danger of *Pseudomonas* infection.

Symptoms	**Diagnosis**	**Treatment**
Pain. Intense photophobia. Tearing.	Topical anesthetic prior to testing for visual acuity. Fluorescent staining and examination with cobalt blue light. Eversion of eyelid to check for foreign body. Examination of cornea and assessment of anterior chamber with slit lamp.	Cycloplegic agent to relieve spasm and pain: cyclopentolate 1%. Erythromycin ophthalmic ointment 4 times daily with or without eye patch if not related to contact lens AND without eye patch if related to organic source. Tobramycin ophthalmic ointment 4 times daily without eye patch if related to contact lens.

Foreign bodies in the eye

Foreign bodies in the eye should be assessed carefully with slit lamp and corneal examination using optical sectioning before attempting removal of the foreign body. Foreign bodies that penetrate the cornea full-thickness should not be removed in the ED, but superficial foreign bodies can safely be removed. Procedure:

- Apply topical anesthetic to both eyes (to suppress blinking in the unaffected eye).
- Hold eye open by hand or with wire eyelid speculum.
- Remove foreign body carefully with small gauge needle or moistened cotton swab.
- Remove iron line (potentially caused by contact with metallic object) with ophthalmic burr (if not over pupil) and refer patient to ophthalmologist for further iron line removal within 24 hours.
- Evert eyelid and examine carefully for further foreign bodies.

- Treat abrasions as indicated.

Foreign body in the ear

Foreign bodies in the ear can be organic or inorganic materials or insects. Careful history should be done to determine the type of foreign body before attempting removal. Children may require conscious sedation or general anesthesia for deep insertions. Irrigations should not be done if tympanic membrane is ruptured or cannot be visualized. Procedure:

- Examine ear to determine if tympanic membrane is intact.
- Drown insects with 2% lidocaine solution and then suction.
- Irrigate small nonorganic particles with pulsatile flow aimed at wall of the canal.
- Use cerumen loops, right-angle hooks, and/or alligator forceps to grasp and remove item.
- Carefully examine the ear canal after removal of the item for lacerations or abrasions.
- Apply topical antibiotic if extensive cutaneous abrasion or laceration or for organic material.

Otitis media

Otitis media, inflammation of the middle ear, usually follows upper respiratory infections or allergic rhinitis. The eustachian tube swells and prevents the passage of air. Fluid from the mucous membranes pools in the middle ear, causing infection. Common pathogens include *Streptococcus pneumoniae*, *Haemophilus influenzae*, and *Moraxella catarrhalis*. Some genetic conditions, such as trisomy 21 and cleft palate may include abnormalities of the eustachian tube, increasing risk. There are 4 forms of otitis media.

Forms	Treatment options
Acute: 1–3 weeks with swelling, redness, and possible rupture of the tympanic membrane, fever, pain (ear pulling), and hearing loss **Recurrent:** 3 episodes in 6 months or 4–6 in 12 **Bullous:** Acute infection with ear popping pressure in middle ear, pain, hearing loss, and bullae between layers of tympanic membrane, causing bulging **Chronic:** Persists ≤3 months with thick retracted tympanic membrane, hearing loss, and drainage	Note: Because 75–90% resolve spontaneously, antibiotics are withheld for 2–3 days. Treatment for persistent infection may include: Amoxicillin for 7–10 days Tympanostomy and pressure-equalizing tubes (PET) for severe chronic or recurrent infections

Otitis externa

Otitis externa (OE) is infection of the external ear canal, either bacterial or mycotic. Common pathogens include bacteria, *Pseudomonas aeruginosa*, *Staphylococcus aureus,* and fungi, *Aspergillus* and *Candida.* OE is often caused by chlorine in swimming pools killing normal flora and allowing other bacteria to multiply. Fungal infections may be associated with immune disorders, diabetes, and steroid use. Symptoms include:

- Pain, swelling, and exudate
- Itching (pronounced with fungal infections)
- Red pustular lesions
- Black spots over tympanic membrane (fungus)

Treatment includes:

- Irrigate ear with Burrows solution or saline to clean and remove debris, foreign objects.

- Bacteria: Antibiotic ear drops, such as ciprofloxacin and ofloxacin. If impetigo, flush with hydrogen peroxide 1:1 solution and apply Bactroban® twice daily for 5–7 days. Lance pointed furuncles.
- Fungus: Solution of 5% boric acid in ethanol; clotrimazole-miconazole solution with/without steroid for 5–7 days
- Analgesics as needed

Foreign body in the nose

Children may insert various organic and inorganic **foreign bodies in the nose**. In most cases, this is observed, but persistent unilateral obstruction of nose, foul discharge, or epistaxis is suggestive of foreign body. Small or uncooperative children may need to be restrained with conscious sedation or papoose board. Procedure:

- Vasoconstrictor/topical anesthetic applied: 1 ml of phenylephrine with 3 ml of 4% Xylocaine®
- Aerosolized racemic epinephrine may be used for decongestion, to loosen foreign body.
- Examine nares with speculum.

Removal techniques:

- Positive pressure: Blowing nose on command. For small children, block opposite nares and have caregiver blow puff of air in mouth, forcing item out of nares.
- Suction with catheter.
- Use alligator or bayonet forceps to grasp item.
- Pass a curette behind item, rotate, and then use to pull item out.
- Insert Fogarty vascular catheter past item, inflate balloon, pull catheter back out.

Recurrent epistaxis

Recurrent epistaxis is common in young children (2–10), especially boys, and is often related to nose picking, dry climate, or central heating in the winter. Incidence also increases between 50–80 years and may be caused by NSAIDs and anticoagulants. Kiesselbach's plexus in the anterior nares has plentiful vessels and bleeds easily. Bleeding in the posterior nares is more dangerous and can result in considerable blood loss. Bleeding from the anterior nares is usually confined to one nostril, but from the posterior nares, blood may flow through both nostrils or backward into the throat and the person may be observed swallowing. People abusing cocaine may suffer nosebleeds because of damage to the mucosa. Hematocrit and hemoglobin should be done to determine if blood loss is significant. Bleeding should stop within 20 minutes.
Treatment:

- Upright position, leaning forward so blood doesn't flow down throat
- Applying pressure below the nares or by pinching the nostrils firmly for 10 minutes
- Severe bleeding: packing and/or topical vasoconstrictors
- Humidifiers may decrease irritation.

Tonsillitis

Tonsillitis is a bacterial or viral infection of the palatine tonsils (lymphatic tissue on posterior pharyngeal wall). Tonsillitis may be acute or chronic. Indications include frequent sore throats, difficulty breathing and swallowing, and enlarged cervical lymph nodes. Sore throats generally persist for >48 hours and may be severe. Tonsils may appear red and swollen and may have purulent exudate. Children may be hoarse and complain of ear pain as well. Fever and chills are common, especially with strep infection, which requires treatment with antibiotics. While no longer done routinely, tonsillectomy may be advised for children who have obstructive sleep apnea because of enlarged tonsils or recurrent tonsillitis (≥3 per year for ≥3 years), although surgery is usually delayed until after 3 years of age because early surgery may stimulate development of other tissue in the nasopharyngeal area.

Surgical Emergencies

Acute abdomen

Acute abdomen is a nonspecific term referring to a child presenting with acute abdominal distress, which could be caused by a number of different disorders. Typical symptoms include abdominal pain, abdominal distention, guarding, rigidity, and fever. Diagnostic procedures usually include a history of medications and treatment; physical exam; complete blood count; and abdominal ultrasound, CT, or MRI, depending on the severity of symptoms. Other lab tests such as renal and liver function tests may be indicated. Infants and children may cry and pull legs to chest. Differential diagnoses for infants include intussusception, volvulus, and congenital defects. Older children and adolescents may have a strangulated hernia, appendicitis, ulcerative colitis, or irritable bowel syndrome. Children with sickle cell disease may be experiencing a crisis. Ketoacidosis may also cause symptoms consistent with an acute abdomen. The primary focus of care is to eliminate possible differential diagnoses.

Incarcerated hernia

Hernias are protrusions into or through the abdominal wall and may occur in children and adults. Hernias may contain fat, tissue, or bowel. There are a number of types that are common in children. Hernias are evident on clinical examination. Incarceration (strangulation) is a life-threatening condition that requires immediate surgical repair.

Indirect inguinal hernias related to congenital defect are most common on the right in males and can incarcerate, especially during the first year and in females.

Umbilical hernias occur in children, especially African American, and rarely incarcerate.

Incisional hernias occur, usually related to obesity or wound infections, and may incarcerate.

Symptoms of incarceration	Treatment
Severe abdominal pain Nausea and vomiting Soft mass at hernia site Tachycardia Fever	Intravenous fluids Immediate surgical excision and fixation Broad-spectrum antibiotics

Hypertrophic pyloric stenosis

Hypertrophic pyloric stenosis (PS) is obstruction of the pyloric sphincter between the gastric pylorus and small intestine, caused by hypertrophy and hyperplasia of the circular muscle of the pylorus so the enlarged tissue obstructs the sphincter. PS is more common in boys than girls and has a genetic predisposition. Onset of symptoms is usually >3weeks. Diagnosis is based on ultrasound. Decreased sodium and potassium levels may not be evident with dehydration.

Signs and symptoms	Treatment

Projectile vomiting (1–4 feet) usually shortly after eating but may be delayed for a few hours. Emesis may be blood-tinged but non-bilious. Infant is hungry and eats readily, but shows weight loss and signs of dehydration. Upper abdominal distention with palpable mass in epigastrium (to right of umbilicus) Visible left to right peristaltic waves	Intravenous fluids to restore hydration and electrolyte balance Surgical pyloromyotomy: longitudinal incisions through the circular muscle fibers down to the submucosa to release the restriction and allow the muscle to expand NPO progressing to enteral feedings postoperatively

Testicular torsion

Testicular torsion is an emergent condition in which the testis rotates, twisting the spermatic cord and impairing circulation with resultant vascular engorgement and testicular ischemia. Testicular torsion is most common in boys 3–20, but it can occur in the neonatal period (70% prenatally). It is commonly associated with the congenital abnormality bell clapper deformity (the testes are situated transversely). In neonates, the testis may be undescended, predisposing it to torsion as it moves. The testis may not adhere adequately to the scrotal wall, so torsion often occurs at 7 to 10 days. Pain is usually acute and the infant cries frantically. The scrotal area begins to swell. The cremasteric reflex (stroking the inner thigh causes retraction of the scrotum/testes) is lost with torsion. Diagnosis is made by testicular scan or sonogram. The torsion must be relieved within 6 hours to prevent further damage. Manual reduction (sometimes effective) or surgical repair is done, with the testis then sutured in the correct position to the lateral scrotum to prevent recurrence.

Ectopic pregnancy

Ectopic pregnancy occurs when the fertilized ovum implants outside the uterus in an ovary, fallopian tube (the most common site), peritoneal cavity, or cervix. Diagnostic studies include vaginal exam, pregnancy test, transvaginal sonography (TVS) to rule out intrauterine pregnancy, HCG titers (increase more slowly with ectopic pregnancy). Progesterone level >22 helps rule out ectopic pregnancy.

Early symptoms	Symptoms of rupture	Treatment
Indications of pregnancy: amenorrhea, breast tenderness, nausea and vomiting. Positive Chadwick's sign (blue discoloration of cervix). Positive Hegar's sign (softening of isthmus). Bleeding may be the first indication as hormones fluctuate. Hormone hCG present in blood and urine.	One-sided or generalized abdominal pain. Decreased hemoglobin and hematocrit. Hypotension with hemorrhage. Right shoulder pain because of irritation of the subdiaphragmatic phrenic nerve.	Methotrexate IM or IV if unruptured and ≤3.5 cm in size to inhibit growth and allow body to expel. Laparoscopic linear salpingostomy or salpingectomy.

Compartment syndrome

Compartment syndrome occurs when muscle perfusion is inadequate because of constriction caused by a cast or tight dressing or because of increase in contents of a muscle compartment as a result of edema or hemorrhage (often related to fractures or crush injuries). It most often affects the forearm and leg muscles. Diagnosis includes clinical examination, Doppler ultrasonography to verify pulses, and tissue pressure measurement (normal is ≤8 mm Hg). Treatment must be initiated immediately to prevent neurovascular damage and necrosis.

Signs and symptoms	Treatment
Severe throbbing pain, unrelieved by opiates. Numbness and tingling as pressure on nerves increases. Cyanosis and decreased or lacking pulse. Edema.	Elevation of affected limb above the heart. Release of constricting cast or dressings. Tissue fasciotomy to relieve constriction if condition is advanced or no response to medical treatment. The wound is left open, allowing the muscle tissue to expand, and covered with moist sterile NS dressing. The limb is splinted and elevated until swelling decreases.

Slipped capital femoral epiphysis (SCFE)

A **slipped capital femoral epiphysis (SCFE)** is an inferior/posterior separation of the ball (proximal femoral epiphysis) of the hip joint from the femur. This separation occurs at the growth plate. A stable SCFE allows ambulation but an unstable does not, even with crutches. Unstable SCFE poses an increased risk of avascular necrosis. SCFE is most common in adolescent boys (2.4 X incidence in girls); especially those who are overweight, have hormonal imbalances, or are experiencing rapid growth. Symptoms include limp, knee pain, lateral rotation of the leg, and stiffness in the hip joint. SCFE most frequently involves the left hip. Patients <10 usually have metabolic disorders, such as hypothyroidism and growth hormone disorders. Acute SCFE has duration of <3 weeks and chronic >3 weeks. Treatment includes internal fixation with best results found if surgery is done within 24 hours of onset or after 48 hours. Because the condition often occurs in the opposite hip as well, some specialists recommend prophylactic fixation, but this remains controversial in the United States.

Tonsillectomy

A **tonsillectomy**, often combined with adenoidectomy, may be performed by a variety of different methods, with some posting more risk of postoperative bleeding than others. Hemorrhage may occur in the initial 24-hour postoperative period (primary) or after 7–10 days (secondary) when the scar begins to slough. Indications of bleeding include evidence of bright red blood in the mouth, spitting up of blood, or excessive swallowing as blood runs down the back of the child's throat. The first indication the child has been swallowing blood may be hematemesis. Bleeding may occur from either the tonsillectomy or adenoidectomy site. Other indications include pallor, restlessness, thirst, hypotension, and tachycardia (>100). Initial treatment includes starting IV line, blood sample for type and crossmatch, and gentle suctioning of large clots. Small bleeding sites or those slowly oozing may be cauterized. The child should sit upright with an ice collar. Uncontrollable bleeding requires immediate surgical intervention with rapid sequence induction. Blood transfusions may be necessary with severe bleeding.

Pediatric fluid deficit

Pediatric fluid deficit must also be carefully estimated and managed. Fluid deficit should be replaced over 3 hours with half of the volume in the first hour and a quarter in each of the remaining 2 hours. Fluid deficit is calculated by first finding the maintenance fluid requirement:Maintenance fluid mL X hours NPO = fluid deficit. Preoperative deficits usually are treated with lactated Ringer's or 1/ normal saline (which may cause hyperchloremic acidosis). Glucose-containing fluids may contribute to hyperglycemia.

Weight in kg	24-hr fluid requirement	Hourly requirement
<10 kg	100 mL/kg	4 mL/kg
10–20 kg	1000 mL and 50 mL/kg for each kg >10 kg	40 mL and 2 mL/kg for each kg >10 kg
>20 kg	1500 mL and 20 mL/kg for each kg >20 kg	60 mL and 1 mL/kg for each kg above 20 kg

Fluid replacement must account for both blood loss and third space loss: Blood: Replacement may be with lactated Ringers (3 mL to 1 mL blood loss) or 5% albumin colloid (1 mL to 1 mL blood loss) to maintain hematocrit at predetermined adequate minimal level. Infants and neonates: >30% (may be as high as 40–50%). Older children: 20–26%

Allowable blood loss is calculated by the following formula based on the child's average hematocrit:
Average hematocrit = (beginning hematocrit + minimum adequate hematocrit) / 2.
Allowable blood loss = [estimated blood loss X (beginning hematocrit – minimum adequate hematocrit)] / average hematocrit.
Blood loss should be monitored carefully to determine when it exceeds the allowable blood loss.
Blood is replaced with packed red blood cells when the allowable blood loss threshold is exceeded.
Volume of packed red blood cell replacement is based on the hematocrit of packed cells, 75%:
Packed red blood cells in mL = [(estimated blood loss – allowable blood loss) X minimum adequate hematocrit] / packed red blood cell hematocrit of 75.
If blood loss is in excess of 1–2 blood volumes, then 10–15 mL/kg of platelets and FFP are administered.

Third space loss can only be estimated based on the degree of trauma related to the surgery:
Minor: 3–4 mL/kg/hr
Moderate: 5–6 mL/kg/hr
Severe: 7–10 mL/kg/hr
Lactated Ringers is most commonly used to replace third space loss

Herniation syndrome

Brain herniation/herniation syndrome occurs when pressure inside of the brain causes a shift in brain tissue from one area of the brain to another (transtentorial), through a surgical opening (extracranial), or through the foramen magnum at the base of the skull. Causes of increased intracranial pressure and brain herniation include hydrocephalus, primary or metastatic brain tumor, trauma, stroke, and abscess. The primary goal of treatment is to control ICP. Treatment may include diuretics (mannitol or furosemide), continuous infusion of hypertonic saline (3%), or invasive procedures, such as burr holes and placing of a ventricular catheter to drain CSF and monitor pressure. If no spinal injury, the head of bed is usually elevated to 30° with head in neutral position. A urinary catheter is inserted so fluid intake and output can be carefully managed and TPN or enteral nutrition started within 72 hours. Severe brain damage or death may occur without prompt recognition and treatment.

Burn injuries

Burn injuries may be chemical, electrical, or thermal and are assessed by the area, percentage of the body burned, and depth.
First-degree burns are superficial and affect the epidermis, causing erythema and pain.
Second-degree burns extend through the dermis (partial thickness), resulting in blistering and sloughing of epidermis.
Third-degree burns affect underlying tissue, including vasculature, muscles, and nerves (full thickness).
Burns are classified according to the American Burn Association's criteria.

Minor	<10% body surface area (BSA) 2% BSA with 3rd degree without serious risk to face, hands, feet, or perineum
Moderate	10–20% combined 2nd–3rd degree burns <10 years ≤10% full thickness without serious risk to face, hands, feet, or perineum
Major	20% BSA; ≥10% 3rd degree burns All burns to face, hands, feet, or perineum that will result in functional/cosmetic defect Burns with inhalation or other major trauma

Complications of burn injuries

Burn injuries begin with the skin but can affect all organs and body systems, especially with a major burn.

- **Cardiovascular:** Cardiac output may fall by 50% as capillary permeability increases with vasodilation and fluid leaks from the tissues.
- **Urinary:** Decreased blood flow causes kidneys to increase ADH, which increases oliguria. BUN and creatinine levels increase. Cell destruction may block tubules, and hematuria may result from hemolysis.
- **Pulmonary/Inhalation:** Injury may result from smoke inhalation or (rarely) aspiration of hot liquid. Pulmonary injury is a leading cause of death from burns and is classified according to degree of damage:
- First: Singed eyebrows and nasal hairs with possible soot in airways and slight edema
- Second: (at 24 hours) stridor, dyspnea, and tachypnea with edema and erythema of upper airway, including area of vocal chords and epiglottis
- Third: (at 72 hours) worsening symptoms if not intubated and if intubated, bronchorrhea and tachypnea with edematous, secreting tissue
- **Multisystem** complications of burn injuries include:
- **Neurological:** Encephalopathy may develop from lack of oxygen, decreased blood volume and sepsis. Hallucinations, alterations in consciousness, seizures and coma may result for recovery is usual.
- **Gastrointestinal:** Ileus and ulcerations of mucosa often result from poor circulation. Ileus usually clears within 48–72 hours, but if it returns it is often indicative of sepsis.
- **Endocrine/metabolic:** The sympathetic nervous system stimulates the adrenals to release epinephrine and norepinephrine to increase cardiac output and cortisol for wound healing. The metabolic rate increases markedly. Electrolyte loss occurs with fluid loss from exposed tissue, especially phosphorus, calcium, and sodium, with an increase in potassium levels. Electrolyte imbalance can be life threatening if burns cover >20% of BSA. Glycogen depletion occurs within 12–24 hours and protein breakdown and muscle wasting occur without sufficient intake of protein.

Management of burn injuries

Management of burn injuries must include both wound care and systemic care to avoid complications that can be life threatening. Treatment includes:

- Establishment of airway and treatment for inhalation injury as indicated:
- Supplemental oxygen, incentive spirometry, nasotracheal suctioning
- Humidification
- Bronchoscopy as needed to evaluate bronchospasm and edema
- β-agonists for bronchospasm, followed by aminophylline if ineffective
- Intubation and ventilation if there are indications of respiratory failure. This should be done prior to failure. Tracheostomy may be done if ventilation >14 days.
- Intravenous fluids and electrolytes, based on weight of child and extent of burn. Parkland formula: 4 ml/kg body weight x BSA per 24 hours.
- Enteral feedings, usually with small lumen feeding tube into the duodenum
- NG tube for gastric decompression to prevent aspiration
- Indwelling catheter to monitor urinary output. Urinary output should be 0.5–2 ml/kg/hr.
- Analgesia for reduction of pain and anxiety
- Topical and systemic antibiotics
- Wound care with removal of eschar and dressings as indicated

Electrical burns

Electrical burns most often occur in children <6, often from biting on a cord. The extent of damage varies widely depending on the site of contact, the voltage, and the duration of contact. Most tissue damage occurs at the point of contact (mouth, head, hands) and the ground contact (feet). In addition to burn injuries, children may have respiratory arrest, ventricular fibrillation, conduction abnormalities, or asystole, seizure, spinal cord injury, compartment syndrome, rhabdomyolysis, and perforated eardrum, so complete assessment is essential. With oral electrical burns, severe damage and ulceration to the mouth may result in eschar and deformity within 2 to 3 days, with increased risk of hemorrhage when eschar sloughs in 2 to 3 weeks. Treatment for electrical burns includes:

- Stabilize ABCs and conduct primary survey.
- IV fluids to maintain urinary output at 0.5 to 1 mL/kg per hour for large burns or evidence of myoglobinuria
- Cardiac monitoring
- Tetanus immunization and wound care as needed
- Referral to burn specialists for all but most minor injuries

Near-drowning

Near-drowning is a common cause of accidents in children, especially in swimming pools. In adolescents and adults, the incidents most commonly occur in lakes, rivers, and the ocean, related to risk-taking and altered level of awareness because of drugs or alcohol. Submersion usually causes aspiration (wet drowning) but may trigger severe laryngospasm (dry drowning).

Laryngospasm sequence	Aspiration sequence
Cardiac arrest with hypoxic/acidosis to brain Decreased oxygen, glucose, and adenosine triphosphate Decreased sodium, potassium pump Increased Na and water in intracranial fluid Cerebral intracellular edema leading to neuronal death	Cardiac arrest with hypoxia/acidosis to other organs (heart, kidneys) Decreased oxygen, glucose, adenosine triphosphate Decreased sodium, potassium pump Increased Na and water in intracranial fluid

	Hypovolemia with shock and death

Submersion asphyxiation can cause profound damage to the central nervous system, pulmonary dysfunction related to aspiration, cardiac hypoxia with life-threatening arrhythmias, fluid and electrolyte imbalances, and multi-organ damage, so treatment can be complex. Hypothermia related to near-drowning has some protective effect because blood is shunted to the brain and heart.
Treatment includes:

- Immediate establishment of airway, breathing and circulation (ABCs)
- High flow 100% oxygen with face mask with intubation if respiratory distress worsens
- NG tube and decompression to reduce risk of aspiration
- Fluid management to prevent/control cerebral/pulmonary edema
- Neurological evaluation
- Pulmonary management includes monitoring for ≥72 hours for respiratory deterioration. Ventilation may need positive end-expiratory pressure (PEEP), but this poses danger to cardiac output and can cause barotrauma, so use should be limited.
- Monitoring of cardiac output and function
- Neurological care to reduce cerebral edema and increased intracranial pressure, and prevent secondary injury
- Treatment of GI stress ulcers and acute renal failure

Head trauma

Head injuries that occur at the time of trauma include fractures, contusions, hematomas, and diffuse cerebral and vascular injury. These injuries may result in hypoxia, increased intracranial pressure, and cerebral edema. Open injuries may result in infection. Patients often suffer initial hypertension, which increases intracranial pressure, decreasing perfusion. Often the primary problem with head trauma is a significant increase in swelling, which also interferes with perfusion, causing hypoxia and hypercapnia, which trigger increased blood flow. This increased volume at a time when injury impairs auto-regulation increases cerebral edema, which, in turn, increases intracranial pressure and results in a further decrease in perfusion with resultant ischemia. If pressure continues to rise, the brain may herniate. Concomitant hypotension may result in hypoventilation, further complicating treatment.
Treatments include:

- Monitoring ICP and CCP
- Providing oxygen
- Elevating head of bed and maintaining proper body alignment
- Giving medications: analgesics, anticonvulsants, and anesthetics
- Providing blood/fluids to stabilize hemodynamics
- Managing airway, providing mechanical ventilation if needed
- Providing osmotic agents, such as mannitol and hypertonic saline solution, to reduce cerebral edema

Infants and small children often exhibit symptoms of **acute head trauma** that are nonspecific or different than the typical symptoms of adults. There may be associated injuries, such as laceration or bruising evident.

- **Mild injuries:** Children may be irritable and restless or somnolent and listless. They may lose consciousness or have periods of confusion. Pallor and vomiting are common.
- **Progressive injuries:** As the condition worsens, alterations of consciousness appear, and children may be difficult to rouse. There may be agitation and marked fluctuations in vital

signs, as well as focal neurological deficits (paralysis, spasticity, paresis, or lack of sensation in one part of the body).
- **Severe injuries:** Children may show signs of increased intracranial pressure, retinal hemorrhage, hemiparesis/hemiplegia or quadriparesis/quadriplegia, thermal deregulation with elevated temperature. Older children may exhibit uncoordinated gait and papilledema.

Complications of head trauma

A variety of different injuries can occur as a result of **head trauma**.

- **Concussions** are the most common injury and are usually relatively transient, causing no permanent neurological damage. They may result in confusion, disorientation, and mild amnesia, which last only minutes or hours.
- **Contusions/lacerations** are bruising and tears of cerebral tissue. There may be petechial areas at the impact site (coup) or larger bruising. Contrecoup injuries are less common in children than in adults. Areas most impacted by contusions and lacerations are the occipital, frontal, and temporal lobes. The degree of injury relates to the amount of vascular damage, but initial symptoms are similar to concussion; however, symptoms persist and may progress, depending upon the degree of injury. Lacerations are often caused by fractures.
- **Skull fractures** are common in adolescents engaged in contact sports, such as football, but may result from severe blunt trauma, as in being in a car accident or being hit with a baseball bat. Symptoms will relate to the location and extent of the fracture, but typical symptoms include:
    - Bruise, swelling, deformity, or laceration at the point of injury
    - Bleeding from nose or ears
    - Clear fluid draining from eyes or ears (cerebrospinal fluid)
    - Pain and tenderness at injury site and more generalized headache
    - Battle's sign—bruising behind the ear—indicates a posterior basilar fracture (delayed sign)
    - Raccoon eyes—bruising and discoloration about the eyes—is a sign of a frontal basilar fracture (delayed sign)
    - Alterations in consciousness or lack of consciousness
    - Pupils unequal
    - Assessment for ABCs should be done first and then neurological assessment. The person should be immobilized while awaiting emergency transfer, as skull fractures may be associated with spinal cord injury.

Spinal cord injury

Spinal cord injury is less common in young children than adults, with the highest incidence between ages 16–30, primarily occurring as the result of automobile or sporting accidents, although shooting and knifing assaults are also implicated. Automobile accidents may cause spinal cord injury even without vertebral fracture if children are not properly restrained. The degree of disability relates to the level of injury. The areas most commonly injured are those with the greatest mobility: 5–7th cervical, 12th thoracic, and 1st lumbar. Damage may vary.

- **Transient** with contusion and bruising with complete recovery
- **Laceration/ compression** with some resultant paresis
- **Transection** with complete paralysis below the area of injury: Paraplegia or quadriplegia

Injuries may be primary with direct trauma to the spinal cord, or secondary as a physiological response to contusion, resulting in ischemia, edema, and hemorrhage that cause destruction of the myelin sheaths and axons. Secondary injuries are often reversible if treated within 4–6 hours.

Spinal cord injuries may result from blunt trauma, falls from a height, various types sports injuries (especially contact sports, gymnastic, diving), and penetrating trauma. Damage results from mechanical injury and secondary responses resulting from hemorrhage, edema, and ischemia. The type of symptoms relate to the area and degree of injury.

Spinal cord injuries	
Anterior cord	The posterior column functions remain so there is sensation of touch, vibration, and position remaining below injury but with complete paralysis and loss of sensations of pain and temperature. Injury to anterior portion of spinal cord usually results from herniated disks, hyperflexion injuries, or damage to the anterior spinal artery. Prognosis is poor.
Brown-Sequard/ lateral cord	The cord is hemisected resulting in spastic paresis, loss of sense of position and vibration on the injured side, and loss of pain and thermal sensation on the opposite side below level of injury. Prognosis is good. Injury to the right or left half of spinal cord usually occurs from transverse hemisection by knife injury or fracture dislocations.

Spinal cord injuries	
Cauda equina	Damage is below L1 with variable loss of motor ability and sensation, and bowel and bladder dysfunction. Injury is to peripheral nerves, which can regenerate so prognosis is better than for other lesions of the spinal cord.
Central cord	Results from hyperextension and ischemia or stenosis of cervical spine, causing quadriparesis (more severe in upper extremities) with some loss of sensations of pain and temperature). Prognosis is good, but fine motor skills are often impaired in upper extremities. The trunk area may suffer incomplete loss of sensation and control, and bowel and bladder control may remain intact.
Conus medullaris	Injury to lower spine (lower lumbar and sacral nerves) causes lumbar pain, loss of sensation in medial thighs, numbness and weakness in legs and feet, unstable ambulation and can result in impotence and lack of bladder control.
Posterior cord	Motor function is preserved but without sensation.
Spinal shock	Injury at T6 or above, results in flaccid paralysis below lesion with loss of sensations and rectal tone, bradycardia, and hypotension.

Immediate assessment is critical for **acute spinal cord injuries** to ensure that treatment can prevent damage by secondary injury.

- Airway support may include suctioning, insertion of oral airway, supplemental oxygen, or endotracheal intubation with mechanical ventilation.
- Hypotension support with intravenous fluids and assessment is necessary to determine if the cause is neurogenic shock or occult hemorrhage.
- Nasogastric tube is used to prevent ileus and aspiration.
- Spinal radiography (CT or MRI) is often needed to determine the degree of spinal cord injury.
- Evaluation for concomitant head injury with neurological exam and CT may be indicated.
- Methylprednisolone (Solu-Medrol®) or tirilazad for 24 hours if started within 3 hours, or 48 hours if started within 3–8 hours, may be of benefit (studies are inconclusive).
- Immobilization prevents further injury.

Autonomic dysreflexia

Autonomic dysreflexia can occur with central cord lesions at or above T6 and can result in encephalopathy and shock if undiagnosed and untreated. Autonomic dysreflexia occurs only after initial spinal shock has resolved. Onset is often very sudden and constitutes a medical emergency.

Common causes include distended bladder, fecal impaction, pressure sores, tight clothing, hyperthermia, and other painful stimuli.

Symptoms	Treatment
Hypertension, severe pounding headache, increased ICP, and/or rupture of cerebral vessel Bradycardia, other cardiac arrhythmias Diaphoresis, piloerection, flushing of skin below level of injury and pallor above Nasal congestion Blurred vision, spots in visual field Seizures	Elevate head immediately to reduce blood pressure. Identify and rectify cause (check bladder, bowels, skin, clothing, temperature). If related to bladder distention, catheterize and drain the bladder slowly. If initial treatment is not successful in reversing symptoms, then give medications (IV antihypertensives, such as hydralazine, and antispasmodics).

Fractures

Fractures and dislocations are commonly diagnosed by clinical examination, history, and radiographs. Careful inspection, observation of range of motion, palpation, and observation of abnormalities are important because pain may be referred. Neurovascular assessment should be done immediately to prevent vascular compromise. Radiographs should usually precede reduction of dislocations to ensure there are no fractures and follow reduction to ensure the dislocation is reduced. Treatment includes:

- Analgesia and sedation as indicated
- Application of cold compresses and elevation of fractured area to reduce edema
- Reduction of fracture: steady and gradual longitudinal traction to realign bone
- Immobilization with brace, cast, sling, or splint indicated
- Reduction of dislocation: varies according to area of dislocation
- Open fracture:
- Wound irrigation with NS
- Tetanus prophylaxis
- Antibiotic prophylaxis
- Referral to orthopedic specialist for open fractures, irreducible dislocations, and complications such as compartment syndrome or circulatory impairment

Fractured ribs

Fractured ribs are usually an indication of severe injury in children because the elasticity of their ribs makes them resistant to fracture. Most fractures are the result of severe trauma, such as blunt force from a motor vehicle accident or physical abuse. Children presenting with rib fractures from "falls" or other vague reports of injury should be examined for signs of abuse and have a radionuclide bone scan that will show both new and old fractures. Since much force is required to fracture a child's ribs, underlying injuries should be expected according to the area of fractures.

- Upper 4 ribs: injuries to trachea, bronchi, or great vessels
- Middle ribs (4–9): pneumothorax or hemothorax from penetration wounds
- Bottom ribs: trauma to liver, kidney, and/or spleen

Treatment is primarily supportive as rib fractures usually heal in about 6 weeks. Underlying injuries are treated according to the type and degree of injury.
Supplemental oxygen. Analgesia. Pulmonary physiotherapy.

Pediatric fractures

Pediatric fractures: Types	
Bend	Children's flexible bones may bend up to 45° without breaking. While they will slowly straighten, they will not do so completely. Bends are most common in ulna with fracture of the radius and in the fibula with fracture of the tibia.
Buckle	When porous bone is compressed, a bulging occurs, usually near the metaphysis. Buckles are most common in younger children.
Comminuted	A comminuted fracture involves bone fragments chipping off from the broken bone and lying in the surrounding tissue. Because children's bones are more pliable than adults, comminuted fractures are rare but may occur in adolescents.
Complete	The bone fragments are completely separated but may be attached on one side by a periosteal hinge.
Greenstick	This is an incomplete fracture on one side of a bone.
Spiral	This spiraling, circular fracture goes around the bone shaft and often results from child abuse.

Fracture of the clavicle

Fracture of the clavicle is the most common pediatric fracture, with some associated with childbirth trauma and half occurring <age 7. There are 3 classes:

- **Middle third of clavicle** (80%): Usually from force on the lateral shoulder related to fall, motor vehicle accident, or sports injury. Treatment includes sling or figure-eight immobilization. Displaced fractures may be surgically repaired.
- **Lateral third** (15%): Usually from force on top of shoulder and may be nondisplaced (type I), displaced (type II) or involving the articular surface of the joint (type III). Treatment includes ice (initially) and sling. Displaced fractures usually require surgical repair.
- **Middle third** (5%): Usually from force against the anterior chest. Treatment includes ice (initially), reduction if displaced, sling, and close observation for intrathoracic injury.

Indications include pain, restricted movement of upper extremity, edema, deformity, and bruising. With compression of nerves or vasculature, circulatory compromise and numbness or weakness may be evident. In rare cases, pneumothorax may occur.

Fracture of the wrist

A **wrist fracture** can occur in the distal radius (thumb side), ulna, or the wrist joint. The radius is the most commonly fractured, but both the radius and ulna may be fractured. Fracture usually occurs from falls with the weight falling on an outstretched hand, resulting in hyperextension, or direct blunt trauma. It is most common in sports such as football, soccer, hockey, skiing, and ice-skating. Pain is usually severe and deformity may be obvious. Mobility is often markedly decreased and the child has an inability to bear any weight on the wrist. Edema often begins immediately, and there may be tingling or numbness as nerves are compressed. Any bleeding should be controlled with compression and dressings applied to open wounds. The bones are aligned and wrist casted or splinted. If both bones are broken, internal fixation may be required.

Elbow dislocation/fracture

Dislocation or fracture of an elbow may present with similar symptoms and radiograph may be needed for diagnosis. The injury usually results from fall or blunt trauma to the elbow. The child complains of severe pain, and muscle spasms may occur. Mobility is limited and there may be obvious deformity. Usually edema begins immediately after injury. There may be pallor and coolness of the arm and hand distal to the injury. The child may exhibit signs of shock. Immediate care includes treating for shock, monitoring pulses, and splinting the elbow. No attempt should be made to change the position of the elbow as it may increase damage to nerves and vessels. It should be splinted as found and ice applied initially. Supracondylar fractures are common in children <8 and epicondylar from 9 to 14. Growth plate fractures may arrest growth. Treatment depends on degree and specific site of injury and may include manipulation, immobilization in sling, cast, or splint or surgical repair.

Fracture of the tibia/fibula

Fracture of the tibia or fibula, or both bones, may occur as a result of a twisting injury at any point from the proximal to the distal ends. The fibula is more protected by tissue, and fracture of this bone alone may be more difficult to detect as the tibia provides a natural splint. There may be little obvious deformity, and the child may be able to walk. Tibia fractures are more likely to result in an open fracture because of proximity to the skin surface. If both bones are fractured, there is usually pronounced deformity and edema at the site of the fractures with severe pain and marked tenderness on palpation. Immediate treatment includes stopping blood flow with compression, monitoring pulses, applying dressing to an open wound, splinting the leg with rigid splints on each side of the leg to prevent the legs from rotating, and parenteral analgesia. Treatment may include immobilization with cast or splint or surgical fixation, depending on site and degree of injury.

Shoulder dislocation

Shoulder dislocations are common injuries resulting from blunt trauma or hyperextension. Usual symptoms include the injured child holding the arm away from the body. (Fractured humerus usually causes the person to hold the arm against the body with the arm across the chest.) There is usually acute severe pain in the shoulder, obvious squaring deformity, and functional loss. There may be numbness or partial paralysis of the arm from compression on nerves or blood vessels. The trainer should not attempt to reduce the dislocation as this could cause further damage. Initially, arm should be supported by placing a pillow or other roll (such as a blanket) between the chest wall and the arm. Then, an arm sling with swathing may be applied to prevent pressure on the joint. Pulses and circulation must be monitored. Procedural sedation and analgesia is usually used for reduction with young children but local intraarticular anesthetic or nerve block may be used in some cases. Radiographs should be taken before and after reduction.

Small cuts and lacerations

When a child gets a **cut or laceration** from blunt or sharp trauma, he or she may react to the trauma by becoming faint; additionally, if there is excessive blood loss, the person may develop shock as the blood pressure falls, so the overall condition and amount of blood loss should be assessed. (Hemorrhage requires immediate emergency treatment.) Pressure should be applied to a bleeding lesion to stop bleeding and then the area thoroughly flushed with soap and water or saline, especially if the wound is contaminated. For small cuts, skin edges should be aligned and Steri-Strips® placed over the wound and a protective dressing should be placed over the cut/laceration. Antibiotic ointment, such as Neosporin®, may be applied to reduce the chance of infection. Suturing may be indicated for large or deep cuts. The child's tetanus immunization record must be checked as the child may require tetanus prophylaxis.

Sprain injuries

A **sprain** is damage to a joint, with a partial rupture of the supporting ligaments, usually caused by wrenching or twisting that may occur with a fall. The rupture can damage blood vessels, resulting in edema, tenderness at the joint, and pain on movement with pain increasing over 2–3 hours after injury. An avulsion fracture (bone fragment pulled away by a ligament) may occur with strain, so x-rays rule out fractures. Sprains may be classified according to severity.

- **1st degree:** This is a relatively mild degree of injury, usually associated with good range of motion and mild pain. Swelling may vary considerably, depending upon whether vessels are disrupted by the sprain.
- **2nd degree:** This comprises a wide range of signs and symptoms, as there is further injury and partial rupture of the ligaments. Usually range of motion is limited by pain. Edema and bruising are usually present but vary in degree. The joint may be somewhat unstable.
- **3rd degree:** This involves total rupture of the ligament with immediate marked pain (although sometimes less than with 2nd degree), bruising, edema, and decreased range of motion. The joint is usually markedly unstable.

Muscle strain: First degree

A **strain** is a overstretching of a part of the musculature ("pulled muscle") that causes microscopic tears in the muscle or tendon, usually resulting from excess stress or overuse of the muscle. Strains may be caused by blunt trauma to a muscle or overstretching related to sports activities, such as field events, football, and soccer. Common sites for strains include the ankle, back, and hamstrings. Neglect of warm-up routines and fatigue may increase risk of strains. Onset of pain is usually sudden with local tenderness on use of the muscle. Strains are classified according to severity of injury.

Muscle strain	
First degree	This injury is relatively mild and symptoms, such as slight discomfort and tenderness to palpation, may be delayed until the following day, as the athlete may be unaware of the injury. Range of motion remains intact.

Muscle strain: Second and third degree

Muscle strain	
Second degree	This injury comprises a wide range of symptoms resulting from stretching or partial tearing of the muscle or tendon. Pain is usually felt on injury with tenderness on palpation and decreased passive and active range of motion, depending upon the site of injury. There may be signs of injury, such as edema and bruising. Pain increases with passive stretching or active contraction of injured muscles.
Third degree	The muscle or tendon is completely ruptured and pain occurs with injury. A defect may be palpable. Often there is extensive edema and bruising from injury to vasculature. While loss of function in affected muscle occurs, strength and loss of range of motion varies according to site of injury.

Traumatic pneumothorax, open pneumothorax, and hemothorax

Traumatic pneumothorax is a lacerating wound of the chest wall, such as a gunshot or knife wound. It can also result from invasive procedures, such as thoracentesis or lung biopsies or from barotrauma related to ventilation or chest surgery. **Open pneumothorax** occurs when air passes in and out, causing the lung to collapse, a sucking sound, and paradoxical movement of the chest wall with respirations. **Hemothorax** is a common complication of traumatic pneumothorax as blood begins to accumulate in the pleural space because of torn vasculature, such as the intercostal vessels or great vessels, or lacerations of lung tissue. In some cases, both air and blood accumulate (hemopneumothorax). Immediate insertion of chest tube or needle aspiration and evaluation of blood loss is necessary. If blood loss continues, surgical intervention to find and control the source of bleeding may be necessary to prevent hypovolemic shock and cardiorespiratory collapse. Autotransfusion may be considered with continued bleeding

Blunt and penetrating acute abdominal trauma

Acute abdominal trauma in children may be blunt (85%) or penetrating (15%). Blunt trauma from motor vehicle accidents, pedestrian injuries (running into traffic), lap belt injury, and sports injuries are common causes of abdominal injury. About 5% of abdominal injuries are related to child abuse, such as punching or kicking a child in the abdomen.

Blunt injuries comprise crush (compression), shear (tearing), and burst (sudden increased pressure) varieties. Because the rib cage in a young child remains elastic, there may be major internal damage from blunt trauma without rib fractures.

Penetrating wounds, on the other hand, may be related to accidental impaling but are almost always related to gunshot wounds (high energy) or knife assaults (low energy). Gunshot wounds tend to cause more extensive damage than stab wounds. Children's organs are larger in proportion to body size than those of adults, so they are more at risk from penetrating wounds.

Splenic injury

The **spleen** is the most frequently injured solid organ in blunt trauma in children because it's not well protected by the elastic rib cage and is very vascular. Symptoms may be very nonspecific. Kehr sign (radiating pain in left shoulder) indicates intraabdominal bleeding and Cullen sign (ecchymosis around umbilicus) indicates hemorrhage from ruptured spleen. Some children may have right upper abdominal pain although diffuse abdominal pain often occurs with blood loss, associated with hypotension. Splenic injuries are classified according to the degree of injury.

- Tear in splenic capsules or hematoma
- Laceration of parenchyma (<3 cm)
- Laceration of parenchyma (>3cm)
- Multiple lacerations of parenchyma or burst-type injury

Treatment may be supportive if injury is not severe; otherwise, suturing of the spleen may be needed. Because children risk infection with splenectomy, every effort (bed rest, transfusion, reduced activity for at least 8 weeks) is done to avoid surgery because the spleen will often heal spontaneously.

Hepatic injury

Hepatic injury is the most common cause of death from abdominal trauma and is often associated with multiple organ damage, so symptoms may be nonspecific. Automobile accidents cause most blunt trauma, but accidents with mountain bikes account for increasing hematomas of the central area of the liver. Neonatal hepatic injuries are often misdiagnosed. Elevation in liver transaminase levels indicates damage that may require CT examination with double contrast. Liver injuries are classified according to the degree of injury.

- Tears in capsule with hematoma
- Laceration(s) of parenchyma (<3 cm)

- Laceration(s) of parenchyma (<3 cm)
- Destruction of 25–75% of lobe from burst injury
- Destruction of >75% of lobe from burst injury
- Avulsion (tearing away)

Almost all hepatic injuries in children (97%) are treated conservatively, primarily because studies show that most hemorrhage stops prior to surgery. Injuries may take 3–12 months to heal with supportive treatment and close monitoring.

Gastric and intestinal injuries

Gastric injuries in children may result in perforation, primarily at the greater curvature. The risk increases if children are injured with a full stomach after eating a meal and suffer a lap belt injury or fall over the handlebars of a bicycle. Perforation results in severe pain, rigid abdomen, and bloody nasogastric drainage with peritonitis developing within hours, so early diagnosis and surgical repair must be done.

Intestinal injuries from blunt trauma are rare in children although contusions and rupture can occur from lap belt injuries. Indications of rupture often appear 24–48 hours later when the child presents with symptoms of peritonitis, such as distention, abdominal pain, absent bowel sounds, leukocytosis, fever, dyspnea, nausea, and vomiting. Prompt antibiotic therapy and surgical repair with peritoneal lavage must be done. The abdominal wound may be left open to heal by secondary intention.

Peritonitis

Peritonitis (inflammation of the peritoneum) may be primary (from infection of blood or lymph) or, more commonly, secondary, related to perforation or trauma of the gastrointestinal tract. Common causes include perforated bowel, ruptured appendix, abdominal trauma, abdominal surgery, peritoneal dialysis or chemotherapy, or leakage of sterile fluids, such as blood, into the peritoneum. Diagnosis is made according to clinical presentation, abdominal x-rays, which may show distention of the intestines or air in the peritoneum, and laboratory findings, such as leukocytosis. Blood cultures may indicate sepsis. Symptoms of peritonitis are those of an acute abdomen.

Symptoms	Treatment
Diffuse abdominal pain with rebound tenderness (Blumberg's sign) Abdominal rigidity Paralytic ileus Fever (with infection) Nausea and vomiting Sinus tachycardia	Intravenous fluids and electrolytes Broad-spectrum antibiotics Laparoscopy as indicated to determine cause of peritonitis and effect repair

Pancreatic injuries

Pancreatic injury can result from motor vehicle or handlebar accidents or assault with impact to the abdominal area, although it is not a common injury. Penetrating injuries (gunshot wounds and stabbings) are more common. Because of the location of the pancreas, impact compresses it against the vertebral column. About 90% of children with pancreatic injury sustain other abdominal injuries as well, making diagnosis difficult. Symptoms may include diffuse abdominal or epigastric pain and well as vomiting of bile. Pancreatic injuries are classified according to degree of injury.

- Contusion, laceration but ducts intact
- Distal transection or injury of parenchyma with ductal injury
- Proximal transection or injury of parenchyma with probable ductal injury
- Combined injury of pancreas and duodenum

CT scans provide the best tool for diagnosis. Surgical exploration and repair of severe damage is the most common treatment. Pancreatitis and diabetes mellitus may be long-term sequelae.

Compartment syndrome

Abdominal trauma with pronounced shock increases risk of **compartment syndrome** for a number of reasons:

- Edema of the intestines because of trauma and surgical manipulation
- Capillary leakage
- Hemorrhage (retroperitoneal)
- Abdominal packing left in place to control bleeding
- IV crystalloid administration

Pressure within the abdomen may begin to rise rapidly if the abdomen is closed, resulting in decreased cardiac output from pressure on the vena cava, increased airway pressures and acute respiratory distress syndrome, decreased urinary output with decrease in renal blood flow and glomerular filtration, and increased central venous pressure resulting in increased intracranial pressure and cerebral edema. Diagnosis is by measurement of intraabdominal pressure (>25 cm H_2O) by Foley catheter or NG tube with pressure transducer or water-column manometry. If risk for compartment syndrome exists, the wound should not be closed. Sudden release of pressure and reperfusion may cause acidosis, vasodilation, and cardiac arrest, so the child should be given crystalloid solutions before decompression.

Nasal fracture

Nasal fracture can result from any type of blunt trauma to the face. Fracture may be overlooked because of edema, so careful examination of the nose with facial injuries is important. Common causes include altercations and sporting injuries. Septal cartilage is often fractured as well as nasal bones.

Signs and symptoms	Treatment for fracture
Edema Pain Crepitation Ecchymosis Deformity Nasal bleeding	Realignment if necessary Analgesia Nasal decongestant Protective covering Packing only for persistent epistaxis

Diagnosis is based on clinical examination and otoscope. Radiographic studies are not indicated unless other facial fractures are suspected. Clear nasal discharge following injury to the face may indicate leaking of cerebrospinal fluid from torn meninges resulting from fracture of cribriform plate. A drop of clear drainage should be placed on filter paper and examined for a clear area around a central stain of blood. If CSF drainage is suspected, the patient should be placed upright, have a CT scan and neurological consult.

Temporomandibular fracture and/or dislocation

Temporomandibular fracture and/or dislocation can occur as a result of trauma, such as a direct blow to the jaw, or chronic disorders. Dislocations may be anterior (most common and often after extreme mouth opening), posterior, lateral, or superior. Diagnosis includes: Complete head, neck, ear, and dental examination. Radiography, such as x-rays or CT, with significant trauma. Tongue blade test: patient bites hard on tongue blade while examiner twists blade, attempting to break it. If fracture, patient opens mouth to release blade

Signs and symptoms	Treatment
Acute pain Dysphagia Difficulty speaking Edema and rigidity of surrounding muscles Inability to open mouth	Short-acting muscle relaxant Narcotic analgesia/conscious sedation Reduction: Patient on chair with head against hard surface Examiner in front of patient places gloved thumbs in patient's mouth, posteriorly over the surface of the mandibular molars. Examiner applies pressure posteriorly and inferiorly. Alternately, examiner stands behind recumbent patient and applies pressure posteriorly and inferiorly.

Maxillary fractures

Maxillary fractures of the face often are associated with significant other trauma because of the degree of force necessary to fracture the maxilla. Three primary types include:
Le Fort I: horizontal (low downward force)
Le Fort II: pyramidal (low or mid maxilla force)
Le Fort III: transverse (force to bridge of nose or upper maxilla)
However, many injuries are a combination with more than one type of fracture. Diagnosis:
Grasping and moving the hard palate back and forth may shift the facial bones.
Complete head, neck, ear, oral, and nasal examination with slit headlamp, suction as needed, nasal speculum, and otoscope
CT scans of face and brain

Signs and symptoms	Treatment
Malocclusion and open bite. Apparent lengthening of face. CSF rhinorrhea (clear nasal discharge). Periorbital ecchymosis.	Stabilize patient and ensure patent airway. Manually disimpact displaced fragments. Obtain pre-injury photograph to guide surgical fixation. Refer to surgeon for fixation.

Orbital fractures

Orbital fractures most often occur with blunt force against the globe causing a rupture through the floor of the orbital bone or a direct blow to the orbital rim, often related to an assault. Injuries are most common in adolescents and young adults. Diagnosis includes: Complete eye (slit lamp) and vision examination. IOP measurement. CT scan.

Signs and symptoms	Treatment
Essentially asymptomatic. Ecchymosis and edema of eyelid. Infraorbital anesthesia from pressure or damage to infraorbital nerve. Decreased sensation of cheek and upper gum on injured side. Diplopia. Enophthalmos (sunken globe).	Usually supportive. Topical steroids for severe edema. Patient advised not to blow nose for several weeks. Surgical repair about 2 weeks after injury when edema has subsided for extensive fracture (≥33% of orbital floor) or enophthalmos >2mm remaining 10–14 days post-injury.

Zygomatic fractures

Zygomatic fracture involves the arch of bone that forms the lateral border of the eye orbit and the bony cheek prominence, most commonly associated with a blow to the lateral cheek from an altercation or accident. Fracture can result in a tilting of the eye and flattening of the cheek, which may be obscured by initial edema. Fracture may be only of the arch or may be a more extensive tripod fracture of the infraorbital rim, diastasis of the zygomaticofrontal suture, and disruption of the zygomaticotemporal arch junction. Diagnosis is by CT scan, which shows the extent of the fracture as well as the amount of displacement. Treatment for tripod fracture is referral to surgeon for open reduction with fixation and exploration and reconstruction of orbit as needed.

Dental fractures

Dental fractures, most commonly of the maxillary teeth, may occur in association with other oral injuries and may be overlooked unless a careful dental examination is carried out. Fractures are classified according to severity of fracture with treatment to prevent further damage and necrosis.

- **Ellis I**: chipping of enamel
- Smooth rough edges
- **Ellis II**: fracture of enamel and dentin with pain on pressure and air sensitivity
- Protect dentin with glass ionomer dental cement and refer to dentist within 24 hours
- **Ellis III**: fracture of enamel, dentin, and pulp with pain on movement, air and temperature sensitivity; blood may be evident
- Protect dentin with ionomer dental cement or calcium hydroxide base and refer to dentist for prompt treatment
- Oral analgesics
- Alveolar/root fracture: Loose tooth and malocclusion, sensitivity to percussion
- Prompt referral to dentist for splinting and/or root canal

Dental avulsions

Dental avulsions are complete displacement of a tooth from its socket. The tooth may be reimplanted if done within 1–2 hours after displacement although only permanent teeth are reimplanted, not primary.
Procedure:

- Tooth can be transported from accident site to the ED in Hank solution, saline, or milk.
- Cleanse tooth with sterile NS or Hank solution, handling only the crown and avoiding any disruption of fibers.
- If tooth has been dry for 20–60 minutes, soak tooth in Hank solution for 30 minutes before reimplantation.
- If tooth has been dry for >60 minutes, soak tooth in citric acid for 5 minutes, 2% stannous fluoride for 5 minutes, and doxycycline solution for 5 minutes prior to reimplantation.
- Remove clot in socket and gently irrigate with NS.
- Place tooth into socket firmly, cover with gauze and have patient bite firmly on gauze until splinting can be applied.
- Apply splinting material and mold packing over implanted tooth and two adjacent teeth on both sides (encompasses 5 teeth).

Distributive shock

Distributive shock occurs with adequate blood volume but inadequate intravascular volume because of arterial/venous dilation that results in decreased vascular tone and hypoperfusion of internal organs. Cardiac output may be normal or blood may pool, decreasing cardiac output. Distributive shock may result from anaphylactic shock, septic shock, neurogenic shock, and drug ingestions.

Symptoms: Hypotension (age-dependent), tachypnea, tachycardia (age-dependent). BP may be lower if patient receiving β-blockers. Skin initially warm, later hypo-perfused. Hyper- or hypothermia (>38ºC or <36ºC). Hypoxemia. Alterations in mentation. Decreased urinary output. Symptoms related to underlying cause.

Treatment: Treating underlying cause and stabilizing hemodynamics: Septic shock or anaphylactic therapy and monitoring as indicated. Oxygen with endotracheal intubation if necessary.
Rapid fluid administration at 20 mL/kg NS (sometimes up to 40 to 60 mL/kg) over 20 to 30 minutes or isotonic crystalloid every 5–10 minutes as needed. Albumin 4 to 5 mL/kg over 30 minutes to maintain cardiac output. Inotropic agents (dopamine, dobutamine, norepinephrine) if necessary.

Multisystem trauma and multi-organ dysfunction syndrome (MODS)

Multisystem trauma is very common in children because of their small size and lack of protective musculature to protect internal organs. Because the rib cage and skull are relatively elastic, severe internal injuries can result without external evidence, such as fractures.

Multi-organ dysfunction syndrome is progressive deterioration and failure of 2 or more organ systems with mortality rates of 45–50% with 2 organ systems involved and up to 80–100% if there are ≥3 systems failing. Trauma patients and those with severe conditions, such as shock, burns, and sepsis, are particularly vulnerable. In children, MODS is frequently associated with sepsis, septic shock, or SIRS. MODS may be primary or secondary.

- **Primary** MODS relates to direct injury/disorder of the organ systems, resulting in dysfunction, such as with thermal injuries, traumatic pulmonary injuries, and invasive infections.
- **Secondary** MODS relates to dysfunction of organ systems not directly involved in injury/disorder but developing as the result of a systemic inflammatory response syndrome (SIRS) as the patient's immune and inflammatory responses become dysregulated.

Procedural Sedation

Rapid sequence intubation (RSI)

Rapid sequence intubation (RSI) is used in the ED to anesthetize and intubate the nonfasting patient requiring emergency surgery. Initial preparation includes inserting 2 intravenous lines and establishing cardiac monitoring, oximetry, and capnography. The patient should be pre-oxygenated (100%) for ≥3 minutes, but without pressure ventilation that may cause aspiration of stomach contents.
Procedure includes:

- Induction agent: thiopental, ketamine, entamide, propofol

- Sellick's maneuver (pressure applied externally with thumb and index finger to cricoid) to close off the esophagus and prevent aspiration
- Muscle relaxant: suxamethonium
- Suction to clear mouth if necessary
- Laryngoscopy to visualize vocal cords
- ETT inserted, cuff inflated, and ETT secured
- Proper placement verified by capnometer or capnograph
- Pressure released from cricoid
- Additional anesthesia: fentanyl, nitrous oxide, and isoflurane

Induction agents and use of additional sedation may vary from one institution to another, but the primary goal is to safely anesthetize and intubate while preventing regurgitation of stomach contents.

Postoperative nausea and vomiting (PONV)

Postoperative nausea and vomiting (PONV) varies with the type of anesthetic agent used. It occurs in about 20–30% of post-anesthesia patients and may be delayed up to 24 hours. Inhalational agents have a higher incidence of PONV than intravenous, and the incidence is lower with epidural or subarachnoid administration although it may indicate the onset of hypotension. PONV correlates with the duration of surgery, with longer surgeries causing increased PONV. If high doses of narcotics, propofol, or nitrous oxide are used, PONV is often a problem. PONV is most common in young females and also relates to menstruation. It is also increased in those with a history of smoking or motion sickness. Some surgical procedures correlate with PONV: strabismus repair, ear surgery, laparoscopy, tonsillectomy, orchiopexy, and gynecological procedures to retrieve ova. PONV may be associated with postoperative pain, so managing pain is an important factor in preventing PONV.

Post-anesthetic respiratory complications

Respiratory complications are the most common in the post-anesthesia period, so monitoring of oxygen levels is critical to preventing hypoxemia.
Airway obstruction may be partial or total. Partial obstruction is indicated by sonorous or wheezing respirations, and total by absence of breath sounds. Treatment includes supplemental oxygen, airway insertion, repositioning (jaw thrust), or succinylcholine and positive-pressure ventilation for laryngospasm. If edema of the glottis is causing obstruction, IV corticosteroids may be used.

Hypoventilation ($PaCO_2$ >45 mm Hg) is often mild but may cause respiratory acidosis. It is usually related to depression caused by anesthetic agents. A number of factors may slow emergence (hypothermia, overdose, metabolism) and cause hypoventilation. It may also be related to splinting because of pain, requiring additional pain management.

Hypoxemia (mild is PaO_2 50–60 mm Hg) is usually related to hypoventilation and/or increased right to left shunting and is usually treated with supplementary oxygen (30–60%) with or without positive airway pressure.

Post-anesthetic cardiovascular complications

Cardiovascular complications are sometimes related to respiratory complications, which may need to be addressed as well. Complications include:

- **Hypotension** is most often mild and requires no specific treatment. It is most commonly caused by hypovolemia and is significant if BP falls 20–30% below normal baseline. A bolus of IV colloid is used to confirm hypovolemia. If severe, then medications, such as epinephrine, may be indicated. Hypotension may occur with pneumothorax, so careful respiratory assessment must be done.
- **Hypertension** usually occurs ≤ 30 minutes after surgery and is common in those with history of hypertension. It may be secondary to hypoxemia or metabolic acidosis. Mild increases usually don't require treatment but medications may be used for moderate (β-adrenergic blockers) or severe (nitroprusside).
- **Arrhythmias** usually relate to respiratory complications or effects of anesthetic agents. Bradycardia may relate to cholinesterase inhibitors, opioids, or propranolol. Tachycardia may relate to anticholinergics, β-agonists, and vagolytic drugs. Hypokalemia and hypomagnesemia may cause premature atrial and ventricular beats.

Electrocardiogram: PQRSTU waves

The **electrocardiogram** records and shows a graphic display of the electrical activity of the heart through a number of different waveforms, complexes, and intervals.

- P wave: Start of electrical impulse in the sinus node and spreading through the atria, muscle depolarization.

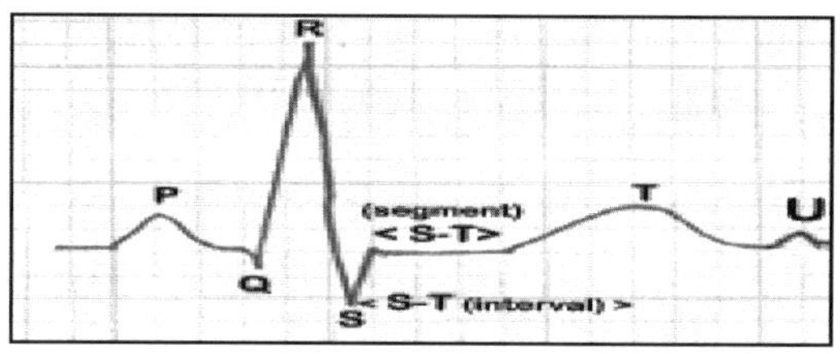

- QRS complex: Ventricular muscle depolarization and atrial repolarization
- T wave: Ventricular muscle repolarization (resting state) as cells regain negative charge
- U wave: Repolarization of the Purkinje fibers. A modified lead II ECG is often used to monitor basic heart rhythms and dysrhythmias:

Typical placement of leads for 2-lead ECG is 3 to 5 cm inferior to the right clavicle and left lower ribcage. Typical placement for 3-lead ECG is (RA) right arm near shoulder, (LA) V_5 position over 5th intercostal space, and (LL) left upper leg near groin.

Blood pressure monitoring

The proper cuff size is necessary for accurate **blood pressure** readings in children. Both standard blood pressure cuffs and electronic blood pressure devices that utilize Doppler or oscillometry techniques can be used. The arm is the most common site for blood pressure readings, but if cuff size is too big, the upper thigh can be used; however, the readings will be 10 to 20 mm Hg higher than readings on the arm. The nurse should refer to standardized charts for boys and girls as BP readings vary widely. The average (50th percentile) for a newborn is 73/55 for boys and 65/55 for girls, and BP slowly increases with age, so the average for a boy at 6 is 96/57 and for a girl 96/57. By age 15, BP is becoming closer to adult level with 114/65 for boys and 111/67 for girls. Both upper and lower extremity blood pressure should be taken one time because a lower pressure in the lower extremity suggests a cardiac abnormality. To estimate normal BP:

- Systolic (ages 1 to 7): Add age in years to 90
- Systolic (ages 8 to 18): Multiply age in years x 2 and add to 83

- Diastolic (ages 1 to 5 years): 56
- Diastolic (ages 6 to 18 years): Add age in years to 52

Pulse oximetry

Pulse oximetry, continuous or intermittent, utilizes an external oximeter that attaches to the child's foot, toe, or finger (depending on age) to indirectly estimate arterial oxygen saturation (SPO_2), the percentage of hemoglobin that is saturated with oxygen. The oximeter also usually attaches to a machine that emits a beep with each heartbeat and indicates the current heart rate and BP. The oximeter uses light waves to determine oxygen saturation (SPO_2). Oxygen saturation should be maintained >95% although some patients with cardiovascular or pulmonary disorders may have lower SPO_2. Results may be compromised by impaired circulation, excessive light, poor positioning, and fingernail polish. If SPO_2 falls, the oximeter should be repositioned, as incorrect position is a common cause of inaccurate readings. Oximetry is often used postsurgically and when patients are on mechanical ventilation. Oximeters do not provide information about carbon dioxide levels, so they cannot monitor carbon dioxide retention. Oximeters cannot differentiate between different forms of hemoglobin, so if hemoglobin has picked up carbon monoxide, the oximeter will not recognize that.

High- and low-flow oxygen delivery

High-flow oxygen delivery devices provide oxygen at flow rates higher than the child's inspiratory flow rate at specific medium to high FIO_2, up to 100%. However a flow of 100% oxygen actually provides only 60–80% FIO_2 to the patient because the child also breathes in some room air, diluting the oxygen. The actual amount of oxygen received depends on the type of interface or mask. Additionally, the flow rate is actually less than the inspiratory flow rate upon actual delivery. Humidification is usually required because the high flow is drying.

Low-flow oxygen delivery devices provide 100% oxygen at flow rates lower than the child's inspiratory flow rate, but the oxygen mixes with room air, so the FIO_2 varies. Humidification is usually only required if flow rate is >3L/min. Much oxygen is wasted with exhalation, so a number of different devices to conserve oxygen are available. Interfaces include transtracheal catheters and cannulae with reservoirs.

Oxygen interfaces

A number of different **oxygen interfaces** are used for the delivery of oxygen to the patient.

Nasal prongs (cannulae)	This is the most common delivery system for oxygen because of ease of use, providing FIO_2 of 24–40% with flows ≤6 LPM. Humidification is needed for flow rates >4 LPM.
Oxygen mask	This covers the nose and mouth, delivering FIO_2 of 30–60%, but flow of oxygen should be maintained between 6 and 12 to prevent rebreathing. Because of the higher flow rate, humidification should be used. Oxygen masks are usually used short-term when higher rates of oxygen are needed.
Venturi mask	Oxygen entrainment masks come with different size color-coded nozzles to more accurately control the FIO_2, with different sizes providing different FIO_2, usually ranging from 24–50% although FIO_2 >35% is not always reliable. Flow rate is 12–15 LPM. Air-entrainment humidifiers may be used to add humidification.

Conscious sedation

Procedural sedation with analgesia (PSA), also referred to as conscious sedation, is used to decrease sensations of pain and awareness caused by a surgical or invasive procedure, such a biopsy, chest tube insertion, fracture repair, and endoscopy. It is also used during presurgical preparations, such as insertion of central lines, catheters, and use of cooling blankets. Conscious sedation uses a combination of analgesia and sedation so that patients can remain responsive and follow verbal cues but have a brief amnesia preventing recall of the procedures. The patient must be monitored carefully, including pulse oximetry, during this type of sedation. The most commonly used drugs include:

- Midazolam (Versed®): This is a short-acting water-soluble sedative, with onset of 1–5 minutes, peaking in 30, and duration usually about 1 hour (but may last up to 6 hours).
- Fentanyl: This is a short-acting opioid with immediate onset, peaking in 10–15 minutes and with duration of about 20–45 minutes.

The fentanyl/midazolam combination provides both sedation and pain control. Conscious sedation usually requires 6 hours fasting prior to administration.

Naloxone

The opioid antagonist, **naloxone** (Narcan®), is similar in structure to agonists, but it displaces agonists at μ receptors (less so at κ or δ receptors). It reverses activity of both endogenous opioids (such as endorphins) and exogenous opioids, such as natural (morphine sulfate) and synthetic (meperidine) opioids, and narcotic antagonist analgesics (such as nalbuphine and butorphanol). It may also serve as an antagonist to the antihypertensive effect of clonidine. Naloxone is primarily used to treat known or suspected narcotic overdose or narcotic depression related to use of narcotics during surgery. Respiratory depression caused by excessive narcotics during surgery usually resolves quickly with naloxone (1–2 minutes), and duration is quite short (30–45 minutes) as the drug is rapidly redistributed, so repeated doses or continuous drip may be needed. If opioid analgesia is abruptly reversed, sympathetic stimulation may occur with resultant tachycardia, hypertension, and pulmonary edema. Withdrawal symptoms may occur in those who are opioid dependent.

Flumazenil

Flumazenil (Romazicon®), a benzodiazepine antagonist, is used for complete/partial reversal of sedation related to benzodiazepine anesthetic induction or maintenance, conscious sedation, or overdose. Treatment (initial dose 0.2 mg or 0.1 mg, pediatric) is given for 15 seconds with a second dose in 45 seconds and at 60-second intervals to 4 doses as needed and then at 20-minute intervals if resedation occurs. Hypnotic effects are usually reversed in <1 minute, but amnesia and respiratory depression may be more persistent. Side effects of reversal include anxiety and withdrawal symptoms in those with long-term use. There may be increased ICP with head injuries. Seizures may be induced if benzodiazepines were used as anticonvulsants or with tricyclic antidepressant overdose. Nausea and vomiting are common. The half-life of flumazenil is shorter than that of benzodiazepines, so in some cases patients are maintained on ventilators until symptoms subside rather than treated with flumazenil.

Consent for procedural sedation and analgesia

Although the child's parents or caregiver sign a general consent for treatment on arrival at the ED, a separate **consent form** should be signed for treatments requiring procedural sedation and analgesia. The consent form should contain the name of the procedure, the purpose of the procedure, and the type of procedural sedation, including agents used. As part of informed consent, the parents or caregiver and child (age-appropriate) should receive a complete explanation of the reason for the procedure and any possible adverse effects of complications. If possible, printed or video information can be provided as well. Additionally, they should receive an explanation of the procedural sedation, the agents used, and possible adverse effects or complications associated with these agents, both in the immediate post-procedure period and possible delayed reactions.

Psychological Emergencies

Suicidal ideation/suicide attempts

Suicide is the third leading cause of death among adolescents with about 1 million attempting suicide in the US each year. Additionally, antidepressants and atypical antipsychotics may increase suicidal ideation and depression.

Suicidal ideation/indications	High risk for repeated suicide attempt
Depression or dysphoria Hostility to others Problems with peer relationships, and lack of close friends Post-crisis stress (divorce, death in family, graduation, college) Withdrawn personality Quiet, lonely appearance, behavior Change in behavior (drop in grades, wearing black clothes, unkempt appearance, sleeping excessively, or not sleeping) Co-morbid psychiatric problems (bipolar, schizophrenia) Drug abuse	Children who actually attempt suicide should be hospitalized and assessed for repeated suicide risk after initial treatment: Violent suicide attempt (knives, gunshots) Suicide attempt with low chance of rescue Ongoing psychosis or disordered thinking Ongoing severe depression and feeling of helplessness History of previous suicide attempts Lack of social support system

Homicidal ideation/attempts

Homicidal ideation or attempts are rare in young children but can occur during adolescence for a variety of reasons.
Sociopathy/psychopathy: These children usually appear quite normal and may even seem charming, but they can be very dangerous because they lack empathy for others. Some are involved in gangs in which violent behavior is expected and valued.

Psychosis: Uncontrolled schizophrenia and paranoia may result in a child behaving in a homicidal manner.

Medications: Medications such as antidepressants, SSRIs, and antipsychotics as well as interferon have been associated with homicidal ideation in some patients. Children on multiple medications may experience an involuntary intoxication that results in rage reactions and sometimes even the death of others.

Children who express homicidal ideation or have attempted homicide require immediate psychiatric referral and may require restraint. The nurse should conduct a complete review of medications and notify security personnel if the child poses a danger.

Schizophrenia

Schizophrenia rarely presents in children and adolescents though it is not unheard of. Many symptoms of schizophrenia mirror normal childhood characteristics and fantasies, so it is particularly difficult to diagnose in this age group. Symptoms of early-onset schizophrenia include:

- Paranoia
- Visual and/or auditory hallucinations
- Bizarre thoughts and beliefs
- Impaired or confused concentration, speech, and social skills
- Inappropriate reaction to events
- Developmental delays

Children with schizophrenia will have disturbances in all settings and are unlikely to show interest in making friends with others. Hallucinations and delusions must persist beyond six months in duration and continue past the age of 7. Early-onset schizophrenia has a very poor prognosis. The client is at high risk for suicide and symptom-related accidental death. Treatment includes antipsychotic medication.

Bipolar disorder

In **children with bipolar disorder**, the hallmark symptom is intense rage. They may experience rage episodes lasting for 2–3 hours. Many parents do not seek treatment for younger children for several years until the child becomes older and the behavior becomes more disruptive. For many younger children, the first symptom exhibited is depression. Symptoms in children under the age of nine usually include labile emotions and irritability rather than more classic manic symptoms. However, as the child becomes older and enters adolescence, the symptoms become more classic-like and include abnormally elevated mood and delusions of grandeur. They may exhibit racing thoughts and pressured speech. Bipolar disease may occur with ADHD, depression, reactive attachment disorder, conduct disorder, and oppositional defiant disorder, so diagnosis and treatment may be complicated. Children often experience academic and behavioral problems as well as suicidal ideation. Initial treatment is monotherapy with a mood stabilizer, such as lithium, carbamazepine, divalproex, or atypical antipsychotics.

Rapid tranquilization for psychotic episodes

A psychotic patient may become extremely agitated. Physical restraints may be required to protect the patient from self-injury or to protect others, but should be followed by chemical restraints in the form of **rapid tranquilization**.
Mild agitation: Lorazepam (Ativan®) 1–2 mg sublingually or by mouth
Moderate agitation: Lorazepam 2 mg and haloperidol (Haldol®) 2–5 mg, OR olanzapine (Zyprexa®) 5–10mg

Severe agitation is usually treated with a combination of drugs and higher dosages:

- Combination 1 mg lorazepam and 5–10 mg haloperidol IM or IV with 1 mg Cogentin® (to counteract dystonia)
- Repeat doses in 20–30 minutes as needed with haloperidol doubled each time up to 20 mg if severe agitation persists.
- Droperidol (Inapsine®) may be substituted in the same dosage as haloperidol. It results in faster sedation, but can cause cardiac abnormalities at high doses (prolonged QT segment).
- Ziprasidone (Geodon®) (10–20 mg IM (usually 20 mg) may be substituted for haloperidol or droperidol if people are sensitive to those drugs. Ziprasidone is often used for younger clients because of lower incidence of dystonia.

Anger, aggression, and violence

Psychological aspects of increased **anger, aggression, and violence** can be associated with uncontrollable instinctual urges or as a result of the child's particular life experiences. Exposure to violence, altered mother/child bonding, altered socialization skills, or reinforcement of aggressive behavior by achievement of a goal can all lead to increased utilization of aggression and violence. Overexposure to violence through the media, entertainment, or immediate environment can possibly lead to a desensitization of aggression and violence and lead to maladaptive behavioral responses. During an assessment, the background history of a child can reveal many different predictors of future maladaptive responses associated with aggression and violence. The history may reveal violent behaviors and rage responses, increasing irritability, or loss of control. Some examples of maladaptive background behaviors include: cruelty to animals or other children, setting fires or other destruction of property, drug or alcohol abuse, self directed violence such as cuts or burns on the arms, or juvenile delinquency. Many of these behaviors are evident during childhood.

Restrictive measures

The use of **restrictive measures** is a last resort in most individual settings. When utilized, restrictive measures are to promote individual safety. The most common type of restrictive measures includes physical restraints and seclusion. Every individual is entitled to being treated with the greatest personal respect and dignity. When an individual's activity is restricted, very careful monitoring is required. Specific documentation on the individual's well being should be performed per the facility's policy and usually includes a description of what occurred that led to restrictive measures and physical monitoring of the individual while in restraints. If restrictive measures have to be utilized, staff members should have attempted and documented any and all other attempts to de-escalate the situation. These restraint techniques should only be utilized during the time that the individual is considered dangerous to him/herself or others.

Chemical restraints

Chemical restraints involve the use of medications, such as lorazepam or haloperidol, to manage an individual's behavior problems. This type of restraint is indicated when individuals are extremely agitated or violent in order to prevent injury to themselves or others. Chemical restraints inhibit individuals' physical movements and make their behavior more manageable. Medication used on an ongoing basis as part of treatment is not legally considered a chemical restraint, which is used only in emergent situations, even though the medications may be the same. There is little consensus about the use of chemical restraints although benzodiazepines and/or antipsychotics are frequently used to control severe agitation. Oral medications should be tried first before injections, as oral medication is less coercive. The trend in psychiatric medicine is to target medications to treat particular symptoms, such as severe agitation, rather than simply to chemically restrain the individual.

Amphetamine and cocaine toxicity

Amphetamine toxicity may be caused by IV, inhalation, or insufflation of various substances that include methamphetamine (MDA or "ecstasy"), methylphenidate (Ritalin®), methylenedioxymethamphetamine (MDMA), and ephedrine and phenylpropanolamine. **Cocaine**

may be ingested orally, IV, or by insufflation while crack cocaine may be smoked. Amphetamines and cocaine are CNS stimulants that can cause multisystem abnormalities. Symptoms may include chest pain, dysrhythmias, myocardial ischemia, MI, seizures, intracranial infarctions, hypertension, dystonia, repetitive movements, unilateral blindness, lethargy, rhabdomyolysis with acute kidney failure, perforated nasal septum (cocaine) and paranoid psychosis (amphetamines). **Crack cocaine** may cause pulmonary hemorrhage, asthma, pulmonary edema, barotrauma, and pneumothorax. Swallowing packs of cocaine can cause intestinal ischemia, colitis, necrosis, and perforation. Diagnosis includes clinical findings, CBC, chemistry panel, toxicology screening, ECG, and radiography.

Treatment includes: Gastric emptying (≤1 hour). Charcoal administration. IV access. Supplemental oxygen. Sedation for seizures: lorazepam 2mg, diazepam 5mg IV titrated in repeated doses. Agitation: haloperidol. Hypertension: nitroprusside, phentolamine 2.5–5mg IV. Cocaine quinidine-like effects: sodium bicarbonate.

Benzodiazepine toxicity

Benzodiazepine toxicity may result from accidental or intentional overdose with such drugs as Xanax®, Librium®, Valium®, Ativan®, Serax®, Versed®, and Restoril®. Mortality is usually the result of co-ingestion of other drugs. Diagnosis is based on history and clinical exam, as benzodiazepine level does not correlate well with toxicity.

Symptoms	Treatment
Non-specific neurological changes: lethargy, dizziness, alterations in consciousness, ataxia Respiratory depression and hypotension are rare complications. Coma and severe central nervous depression are usually caused by co-ingestions.	Gastric emptying (<1 hour) Charcoal Concentrated dextrose, thiamine and naloxone if co-ingestions suspected, especially with altered mental status Monitoring for CNS/respiratory depression, Supportive care Flumazenil (antagonist) 0.2 mg each minute to total 3 mg may be used in some cases but not routinely advised because of complications related to benzodiazepine dependency or co-ingestion of cyclic antidepressants. Flumazenil is contraindicated in the presence of increased intracranial pressure.

Rohypnol ingestion

Rohypnol® (flunitrazepam) is a type of benzodiazepine, commonly referred to as the "date rape drug" or "roofie" because it causes anterograde amnesia. Rohypnol® is popular with teens and young adults and is often taken with alcohol, which potentiates its effects. Rohypnol® is a CNS depressant that causes muscle relaxation, slurs speech and reduces inhibitions. The effects occur within 20–30 minutes of ingestion but may persist 8 to 12 hours. Repeated use can result in aggressiveness, and withdrawal may cause hallucinations and seizures. Overdoses cause hypotension, altered mental status, vomiting, hallucinations, dyspnea, and coma. Diagnosis is by history, clinical examination, and drug testing. Treatment includes:

- Assessment for rape and rape kit if indicated with tests for STDs
- Gastric emptying (<1 hour)
- Charcoal
- Monitoring for CNS/respiratory depression
- Supportive care
- Flumazenil (antagonist) 0.2 mg each minute to total 3 mg may be used in some cases but not routinely advised because of complications related to benzodiazepine dependency or co-ingestion of cyclic antidepressants.
- Counseling referral for rape

Ethanol overdose

Ethanol overdose affects the central nervous system as well as other organs in the body. Ethanol is absorbed through the mucosa of the mouth, stomach, and intestines, with concentrations peaking in about 30–60 minutes. Young children often ingest alcohol in products (perfumes, cleaning solutions) that are more toxic than alcoholic beverages. The liver clears ethanol more rapidly than in adults, at about 30 mg/dL/hr or about 0.5 ounce/hr.

Signs and symptoms	Treatment
Infants/young children: Seizures and coma. Respiratory depression and hypoxia. Hypoglycemia (especially infants and toddlers). Hypothermia. **Adolescents:** Altered mental status. Hypotension. Bradycardia with arrhythmias. Respiratory depression and hypoxia. Cold, clammy skin or flushed skin (from vasodilation). Acute pancreatitis with abdominal pain. Lack of consciousness. Circulatory collapse, death.	Monitor arterial blood gases and oxygen saturation. Ensure patent airway with intubation and ventilation if necessary. Intravenous fluids. Dextrose to correct hypoglycemia. Maintain body temperature (warming blanket). Dialysis in severe cases.

Indicators of substance abuse

Indicators of substance abuse	
Physical signs	**Other signs**
Needle tracks on arms or legs Burns on fingers or lips Pupils abnormally dilated or constricted, eyes watery Slurring of speech, slow speech Lack of coordination, instability of gait Tremors Sniffing repeatedly, nasal irritation Persistent cough Weight loss Dysrhythmias Pallor, puffiness of face	Odor of alcohol/marijuana on clothing or breath Labile emotions, including mood swings, agitation, and anger Inappropriate, impulsive, and/or risky behavior Lying Missing appointments Difficulty concentrating/short term memory loss, disoriented/confused Blackouts Insomnia or excessive sleeping Lack of personal hygiene

Post-traumatic stress disorder

Post-traumatic stress disorder (PTSD) is an anxiety disorder that develops as a response to a severe emotional or physical trauma. The patient is typically numb at first but later has symptoms that may include excessive irritability, nightmares, flashbacks to the traumatic scene and overreactions to sudden noises. PTSD typically develops after a terrifying ordeal that involved physical harm or the threat of physical harm, such as assault, rape, serious accidents, abuse and natural disasters. Feelings common to these traumatic experiences include:

- Overpowering terror, helplessness and fear of being killed
- Recurrent intrusive thoughts of trauma in dreams, during awake periods or through persistent flashbacks
- Avoidance of thoughts or recollections about the trauma
- Avoidance of persons or situations that provoke the memory of the original trauma
- Diminished interest in activities or persons
- Increased startle reflex, sleep disturbances, outbursts of temper, and difficulty concentrating

Child Maltreatment Emergencies

Infant abuse

Infants are especially vulnerable to **abuse**. Healthcare providers should be on alert for indications of abuse.

- Any fracture in a child <2, especially spiral fractures, rib fractures, multiple fractures (which may result from excessive squeezing of the child's chest to quiet the child), and skull fractures (which rarely occur from falls of <1 meter)
- Metaphyseal fractures (ends of long bones) result from grabbing and twisting of extremities
- Scald or burn injuries
- Injuries inconsistent with explanation
- Nonresponsive, listless, or lethargic infant
- Patterns of bruising suggestive of handprint or weapon (such as a belt), especially on the cheek or buttocks. Right handed parents typically strike the left side of the infant's face; and left handed, the right side.
- Bruises of varying duration (yellow to purple to red)
- Bruises in areas other than over bony prominences (the usual site of bruising from normal falls, accidents)
- Injured outer ear (from twisting or striking the child on the side of the face)
- Malnourished infant

Shaken baby/shaken impact syndrome

Shaken baby syndrome is believed to be the result of vigorous shaking of an infant, causing acute subdural hematoma with subarachnoid and retinal hemorrhages. It is believed that the shaking of the brain causes both coup and contrecoup damage as well as damaging vessels and nerves with resultant cerebral edema. Some authorities, however, believe that the extent of injuries typically seen with these infants precludes just shaking and that they must also suffer blunt impact, as the injuries are more compatible with the head striking against a solid surface with great force, so shaken impact syndrome includes shaking AND impact. The American Academy of Pediatrics now recommends the term **abusive head trauma**. Symptoms include:

Subdural (most common) and Subarachnoid hemorrhages. Diffuse brain injury. Bruises and/or Fractures (ribs and extremities). Retinal hemorrhage (common with shaking injuries). Severe residual problems that may include vision and hearing defects, seizures, mental retardation or impaired cognition, paralysis, or coma. Sometimes children may not exhibit obvious neurological symptoms immediately after trauma but have learning disabilities and behavioral disorders that appear in school.

Munchausen syndrome by proxy

Munchausen syndrome by proxy is a disorder in which a caregiver fabricates signs and symptoms of an illness or actively causes illness in a child in order to gain attention of healthcare providers. In most cases (90%) the perpetrator is the mother and the victim an infant (usually <1 year) although some cases involve a young child (≤6). The child often has a history of repeated visits to different physicians, multiple illnesses, repeated invasive procedures to determine the cause of the reported symptoms, and nonresponse to medications and treatment. The symptoms most commonly reported by the caregiver include apnea, diarrhea, fever, seizures, vomiting, rashes, and bleeding (stool, urine). The caregiver may overdose children on medications, prescription and OTC, or give the child ipecac. Perpetrators often have some knowledge of healthcare and may suggest procedures. Confirmation often requires multidisciplinary cooperation. Suspicion of Munchausen syndrome by proxy should result in referral to child protective services.

Physical and emotional abuse

Types of child abuse	
Physical	Indications include beating, striking, scalding, burning, drugging, or withholding medications and/or treatments. Bruises may be in various stages of healing. Multiple fractures or evidence of previous healed fractures may be seen on radiograph. Burns are often in glove or stocking distribution. Ligature marks from being tied may be evident on wrists and ankles.
Emotional	Indications include shaming, threatening, insulting, or embarrassing the child. In some cases, the child's toys or belongings are taken away or destroyed or animals are given away or killed in order to frighten or control the child. Verbal abuse, such as screaming insults or obscenities, is common. Parents/caregivers may make statements, such as "You were a mistake" or "I wish you'd never been born." Emotional neglect occurs when the parents/caregivers are cold and uncaring, showing the child little or no affection.

Sexual abuse

Indications include vaginal discharge, bloodstains on undergarments, genital irritation, STIs, bedwetting, seductive behavior, constant masturbation, and fear of strangers or particular people or places. Sleeping patterns may be disrupted with fear of falling asleep or nightmares. Children may exhibit sudden changes in behavior, such as withdrawal, and develop somatic complaints, such as headaches or stomach aches. Children may develop ongoing feelings of shame, guilt, low self-esteem and anger, and are at increased risk of substance abuse problems, especially as they enter adolescence. Factors associated with severity of psychological problems include abuse over a long period of time, abuse associated with violence or threats, abuse that includes vaginal or anal penetration, and incest (especially involving the father or stepfather. Sexual abuse may occur to both males and females.

Rape and sexual abuse

Rape and sexual abuse victims (both male and female) should be treated sensitively and questioned privately. Examination should include:

- **Assault history** that includes what happened, when, where, and by whom. Questioning should determine if there is a possibility of drug-induced amnesia or activities, such as douching or showering, which might have destroyed evidence.
- **Medical history** to determine if there is a risk of pregnancy and when and if the last consensual sex occurred that might interfere with laboratory findings.
- **Physical examination** should include examination of the genitals, rectum, and mouth. The body should be examined for bruising or other injuries. Toluidine dye should be applied to the perineum before insertion of a speculum into the vagina to detect small vulvar lacerations.

Forensic evidence must be collected within 72 hours and requires informed consent and the use of a rape kit. Forensic evidence includes:

- Victim samples for control
- Assailant-identifying samples
- Evidence of sexual activity

- Evidence of force or coercion

Legal and Professional Issues

Legal Issues

Informed consent

Parents/guardians of children must provide **informed consent** for all treatment the child receives. This includes a thorough explanation of all procedures and treatment and associated risks. Parents/guardians should be apprised of all options and allowed input on the type of treatments. Parents/guardians should be apprised of all reasonable risks and any complications that might be life threatening or increase morbidity. The American Medical Association has established guidelines for informed consent: Explanation of diagnosis. Nature and reason for treatment or procedure. Risks and benefits. Alternative options (regardless of cost or insurance coverage). Risks and benefits of alternative options. Risks and benefits of not having a treatment or procedure. Providing informed consent is a requirement of all states.

Forensic evidence and chain of custody

Emergency nurses come in contact with cases involving **forensic evidence** daily, but much evidence is destroyed, washed or brushed away, contaminated, or overlooked. Each facility should have protocols in place for obtaining and securing forensic evidence, and staff members should be trained. Typical items related to forensic evidence include, hairs, fibers, bullets, and clothing (blood stains, semen stains) as well as fragments of different materials, such as wood, paint, metal, or glass. Nurses should always maintain a level of suspicion when the clinical picture suggests criminal or civil liability. Evidence should be obtained properly and secured in a locked drop box or space with dispensation documented and not disturbed until retrieved by proper authorities in order to maintain the chain of custody. **Chain of custody** refers to the documented record of acquiring, securing, and transferring evidence. This record must contain a chronological paper trail that clearly outlines where and in whose custody evidence is at all times.

Forensic evidence

Forensic evidence	
Clothing	If necessary to cut clothing, try to do so at seams and avoid cutting through any tears, holes, or stains. Remove all clothing carefully without shaking, fold, and immediately secure each piece in a separate paper bag (not sealed in plastic). Wet clothes should be left open to dry or authorities notified immediately.
Bullets	Retrieve bullets with rubber tipped instrument and avoid contact with any metal surface, wrap in cotton, and place in secure container. If sent to pathology department, advise pathology of need to maintain chain of custody and avoid altering the surface.
Weapons	Retrieve knives or other penetrating weapons, using care not to disturb potential fingerprints. Do not wash away blood or other evidence.
Gunpowder particles	If necessary, retrieve particles on skin (such as hands) by swabbing with cotton swab or adhesive applicators and secure.
Statements	Record relevant exact statements the victim or others make.
Wounds	If protocol permits, photograph wounds and bruises. Thoroughly document all wounds and types of bruises, including size, condition, color, shape, and location.

ABCs of forensic nursing (McCracken)

The ABCs of forensic nursing, developed by McCracken, provide a simple mnemonic device to help the nurse remember the steps to carry out in order to obtain forensic evidence.

- **A-Assess** the victim.
- **B**-Serve as a **bridge** or liaison between the facility and outside agencies, such as the police and ME.
- **C**-Maintain the **chain** of custody by following established protocols in obtaining and securing evidence.
- **D-Document** observations, actions.
- **E**-Obtain **evidence.**
- **F**-Provide information to **families.**
- **G-Go** to court as necessary to provide testimony.
- **H**-Learn **hospital** policies and protocols and know how and where to access them if necessary.
- **I**-Maintain a healthy **index** of suspicion and awareness of typical injuries associated with abuse and violent actions.

Emergency Medical Treatment and Active Labor Act (EMTALA)

The Emergency Medical Treatment and Active Labor Act (EMTALA) is designed to prevent patient "dumping" from emergency departments (ED) and is an issue of concern for risk management, requiring staff training for compliance.

- Transfers from the ED may be intrahospital or to another facility.
- Stabilization of the patient with emergency conditions or active labor must be done in the ED prior to transfer, and initial screening must be given prior to inquiring about insurance or ability to pay.
- Stabilization requires treatment for emergency conditions and reasonable belief that, although the emergency condition may not be completely resolved, the patient's condition will not deteriorate during transfer.
- Women in the ED in active labor should deliver both the child and placenta before transfer.
- The receiving department or facility should be capable of treating the patient and dealing with complications that might occur.
- Transfer to another facility is indicated if the patient requires specialized services not available intrahospital, such as to burn centers.

Professional Issues

Ethical and clinical conflict resolution

Ethical and clinical conflicts among patients and their families and healthcare professionals are not uncommon. Issues frequently relate to medications and treatment, religion, concepts of truth-telling, lack of respect for patient's autonomy, and limitations of managed care or incompetent care. Additionally, healthcare providers are in a position to easily manipulate patients/families by providing incomplete information to influence decisions, and this can give rise to ethical conflicts. Facilitation involves questioning and listening, acknowledging each person's perspective while sharing different viewpoints.

Open communication is critical to solving conflicts. Asking what steps could be taken to resolve the conflict or how it could be handled differently often leads to compromise because it allows for exchange of ideas and validates legitimate concerns. Sharing cultural perspectives can lead to better understanding.

Advocacy for the patients/families must remain at the center of conflict resolution.

Patient and family rights and responsibilities

Empowering patients and families to act as their own advocates requires they have a clear understanding of their **rights and responsibilities**. These should be given (in print form) and/or presented (audio/video) to patients and families on admission or as soon as possible.
Rights should include competent, nondiscriminatory medical care that respects privacy and allows participation in decisions about care and the right to refuse care. They should have clear understandable explanations of treatments, options, and conditions, including outcomes. They should be apprised of transfers, changes in care plan, and advance directives. They should have access to medical records information about charges.

Responsibilities should including providing honest and thorough information about health issues and medical history. They should ask for clarification if they don't understand information that is provided to them, and they should follow the plan of care that is outlined or explain why that is not possible. They should treat staff and other patients with respect.

Patient's rights (JC/NCQA)

Patients' (families') rights in relation to what they should expect from a healthcare organization are outlined in both standards of the Joint Commission and National Committee for Quality Assurance. Rights include:

- Respect for patient, including personal dignity and psychosocial, spiritual, and cultural considerations
- Response to needs related to access and pain control
- Ability to make decisions about care, including informed consent, advance directives, and end of life care
- Procedure for registering complaints or grievances
- Protection of confidentiality and privacy
- Freedom from abuse or neglect
- Protection during research and information related to ethical issues of research
- Appraisal of outcomes, including unexpected outcomes
- Information about organization, services, and practitioners
- Appeal procedures for decisions regarding benefits and quality of care
- Organizational code of ethical behavior
- Procedures for donating and procuring organs/tissue

Critical incident stress management

Critical incident stress management (CISM) is a procedure to help people cope with stressful events, such as disasters, in order to reduce incidence of post-traumatic stress syndrome.
Defusing sessions usually occur very early, sometimes during or immediately after a stressful event, and are used to educate personnel who are actively involved about what to expect over the next few days and to provide guidance in handling feelings and stress.

Debriefing sessions usually follow in one to three days and may be repeated periodically as needed. These sessions may include people who were directly involved as well as those indirectly involved. People are encouraged to express their feelings and emotions about the event. Critiquing the event or attempting to place blame is not productive as part of the CISM process.

Follow-up is done at the end of the process, usually after about week, but this can vary.

Promotion of safety and health/wellness in the community

The pediatric emergency nurse is in a unique position to **promote safety and health/wellness in the community** regarding health promotion and disease prevention. There are many avenues that the nurse can explore.

Schools and universities present many opportunities, from demonstrating safety practices, such as wearing bicycle helmets, to small children in elementary school, to speaking with students in medical fields, to giving lectures on health care in university classes or public seminars.

Service organizations often invite speakers to discuss topics of interest, and this presents an opportunity to discuss health issues and to enlist the aid of other organizations in spreading information.

News media is especially interested in information during times of outbreaks or specific health concerns, but they may also be willing to interview or allow reports on a regular basis.

Job fairs present an opportunity to speak to a wide range of people about the health.

Unions may be interested in field-related information about health matters.

Practice Test

Practice Questions

1. During the Pediatric Assessment Triangle, the ER nurse begins by doing which of the following:
    a. Reassure the child with gentle touch
    b. Observe skin color to assess circulation
    c. Note position, chest movement, and ease of breathing
    d. B and C

2. What is the purpose of the Pediatric Assessment Triangle?
    a. Determine the severity of the child's condition
    b. Establish the diagnosis
    c. Verify the level of necessity for further intercession
    d. A and C

3. Upon your initial assessment of a 5-year-old boy, you immediately note that he is cyanotic, breathing rapidly, and assuming the sniffing position. The next step you take is the following:
    a. Begin rapid assessment of airway, breathing, and circulation
    b. Reassure him and encourage him to lie flat
    c. Take thorough history
    d. Perform a comprehensive physical

4. What is the TICLS Assessment used to evaluate?
    a. Respirations
    b. Circulation
    c. Appearance
    d. Temperature

5. A young mother enters the ER with her infant whose head is tilting forward with exhalation and returning upright on inhalation. What is the term for this breathing abnormality?
    a. Sniffing
    b. Head bobbing
    c. Nasal flaring
    d. Gasping

6. A 5-year-old child with a large laceration and extensive bleeding from his lower arm comes into the ER. You immediately apply pressure to the wound. What other first aid do you administer to control the bleeding?
    a. Elevate the arm
    b. Establish cause of injury
    c. Check blood pressure
    d. Start IV

7. What is the maximum single subcutaneous or intramuscular dose of epinephrine for anaphylaxis?
   a. 0.5 mL of 1:1000 solution
   b. 0.1 mL of 1:10,000 solution
   c. 0.3 mL of 1:1000 solution
   d. 5 mL of 1:1000 solution

8. Emergency Nurses Association suggests the use of a mnemonic, CIAMPEDS, when ascertaining the patient history. What does the letter "C" reference?
   a. Contagion
   b. Chief complaint
   c. Circulation
   d. Congenital abnormalities

9. When performing the physical examination during the secondary survey, the inspection and palpation of each section of the body may be necessary using DCAP-BLS-TIC. What does the DCAP portion of this mnemonic reference?
   a. Deformities, Contusions, Abrasions, Penetrations
   b. Delusions, Concussions, Apprehension, Psychosis
   c. Dyspnea, Capillary refill, Appearance, Pallor
   d. Disability, Circulation, Airway, Pulse

10. A 4-year-old boy presents in the ER with confusion, fever, drooling, and difficulty swallowing. As the triage nurse, how do you classify his condition?
   a. His condition is urgent, so he requires attention within 30 to 60 minutes
   b. His condition is emergent, so he requires attention within 10 minutes
   c. His condition is non-urgent, so he can wait up to 2 hours
   d. His condition is semi-urgent, so he can wait 1 to 2 hours

11. You admit an infant who has a history of inconsolable crying for the last several hours. During the physical assessment, you notice a bluish coloration around the umbilicus. What is this sign and what does it indicate?
   a. Kehr sign indicating possible blood irritating the diaphragm
   b. Cullen sign indicating possible blood in the abdomen
   c. Purpura indicating possible vascular defect
   d. Petechiae indicating possible infection

12. Several people accompany a 4-year-old girl to the ER. When asking questions regarding her history, which of the following statements is accurate?
   a. Anyone accompanying the child may answer
   b. Only family members or legal guardians may answer
   c. Only the mother may answer
   d. If a family member or legal guardian is not present, you must contact them by phone

13. In addition to pertinent past medical history, what other information is necessary when assessing an infant or toddler?
   a. Blood type
   b. Sibling's history
   c. Birth information
   d. Allergies to drugs

14. What is the acronym OPQRST used to assess?
   a. Breathing
   b. History
   c. Pain
   d. Circulation

15. Establishing a complete history of prescription medications is an important step in taking the history of a child. What additional information is important?
   a. Expiration dates, brands
   b. Route, dose, frequency, indication, OTC drugs
   c. Manufacturer, generic equivalent
   d. Pharmacy, number of refills

16. When meeting with the family of the patient, what observations regarding their interpersonal relationships are relevant?
   a. Determine the primary caregiver
   b. Assess coping abilities
   c. Determine family dynamics
   d. All of the above

17. Intraosseous infusion (IOI) is a procedure in which medications, blood products, and fluids infuse into the bone marrow cavity. Which of the following is accurate regarding the use of this technique?
   a. IOI absorption is slower than subcutaneous injection
   b. IOI absorption is faster than IV infusion
   c. Must be administered by physician or nurse anesthetist
   d. Blood samples for laboratory testing are possible

18. Which patient requires infant paddles for defibrillation?
   a. 1 year old or 10 kg
   b. 6 month old or 8 kg
   c. 24 months old or 14 kg
   d. 18 months old or 12 kg

19. Application of a conduction material such as gel or paste prior to applying defibrillation paddles helps the current to pass between the pads and the body surface. Which statement regarding defibrillation is accurate?
   a. Damp skin improves current absorption
   b. Wrong paste or gel may cause sparks or fire
   c. Inadequate gel may result in arcing
   d. Excessive gel may result in burns

20. Your unstable patient will require IV therapy for an extended amount of time, with the administration of large volumes of solutions. Peripheral veins are not readily accessible, so which alternative site is indicated?
 a. Frontal scalp vein
 b. Cephalic vein
 c. Central venous
 d. Jugular vein

21. You admit a 5-year-old girl who had experienced a fall and presents with a possible cervical spine and brain injury. She is confused and combative. Which of the following responses is preferable?
 a. You forcibly restrain her to prevent further injury
 b. Enlist the parent or caregiver to hold her in a neutral position
 c. Allow her to move at will
 d. Use sand bags or IV bags to stabilize her neck

22. Chemical injury to the throat occurs when a child consumes caustic material. What is the best first response in treating a child who has ingested a chemical?
 a. Attempt to obtain precise neutralizing agent
 b. Immediately contact poison control before treatment
 c. Wear protective clothing
 d. Flush external chemical burns with copious amounts of water

23. A 7-year-old boy presented in the ER complaining of a severe headache and vomiting. The parents state that he had been playing baseball, and a ball hit him in the temple. Which of the following signs or symptoms indicate increased intracranial pressure?
 a. Tachycardia, irregular respirations
 b. Decreased pulse pressure readings
 c. Bradycardia, pupil changes
 d. Clear nasal discharge

24. Frantic parents bring their 11 month old into the ER and exclaim that he choked on a penny and they cannot dislodge it. You assess the infant and realize that he is conscious but unable to exchange air. What is your first response?
 a. Place the infant face down over 1 arm
 b. Using the heel of your hand, perform 5 back blows between the shoulder blades
 c. Perform 5 chest thrusts 1 finger width below the nipple line
 d. Perform head tilt and jaw thrust

25. What is the condition in which the heart and major blood vessels move to the side of the chest that is opposite an open chest injury?
 a. Tracheal deviation
 b. Mediastinal shift
 c. Simple pneumothorax
 d. Tension pneumothorax

26. Asthma (reactive airway disease) is the most prevalent of the pediatric chronic diseases. When a child comes into the ER with respiratory arrest imminent, which signs or symptoms would you expect to observe?

a. Agitation, tachycardia
b. Loud expiratory wheezing
c. Absence of wheeze, bradycardia
d. Pulsus paradoxus

27. Upon admitting a child with mild symptoms of reactive airway disease, which of the following would be an unacceptable intervention?

a. Application of pulse oximetry
b. Insert IV
c. Allow child to assume a comfortable position
d. Administer oxygen in a manner that does not agitate child

28. What is the most important diagnostic tool for assessing a child who has experienced a seizure?

a. Physical examination
b. History
c. Presence of fever
d. Postictal confusion

29. A young couple brings their recently discharged newborn daughter to the ER. During the examination of the newborn, you notice distention of her abdomen and lethargy. The parents disclose that the newborn was premature and has had bloody diarrhea, poor appetite, vomiting, and a fever, and while in the neonatal nursery had received blood transfusions. What is the most likely condition you suspect?

a. Necrotizing enterocolitis
b. Intussusception
c. Intestinal obstruction
d. Infant acid reflux

30. An 11-year-old boy presents in the ER with swelling of the face, ankles, and feet. His urine specimen appears brown and foamy. What condition do you suspect?

a. Dehydration
b. Kidney disease
c. Heart disease
d. Urethral obstruction

31. There are approximately 450,000 reported cat bites annually. What makes this type of injury so difficult to treat?

a. Avulsion of tissue
b. Bone penetration
c. Deep punctures
d. Penetration of the skull

32. A family enters the ER concerned that their son has eaten wild mushrooms on a camping trip and now has complaints of watery diarrhea and vomiting. What instructions do you give the parents?
   a. Keep him on clear liquids until the symptoms disappear
   b. Try OTC antidiarrheal medications and clear liquids or Gatorade
   c. Explain that he may have serious complications and inquire about type of mushroom ingested
   d. Explain that most mushrooms are nonpoisonous, so they can take him home and monitor him

33. A 7-month-old African American infant arrives in the ER with edema of the hands. Upon physical examination, you palpate the spleen and find it enlarged. What disease process do you suspect?
   a. Mononucleosis
   b. Lymphoma
   c. Kidney disease
   d. Sickle cell anemia

34. A 12-year-old boy comes into the ER holding an ice bag to his eye. His parents inform you that he sustained an injury to the eye from a baseball. Upon examination, you note blood in the anterior chamber of the eye. Which of the following do you suspect?
   a. Conjunctivitis
   b. Detached retina
   c. Hyphema
   d. Cataract

35. You admit a 14 year old who has recently received chemotherapy for acute lymphoblastic leukemia. He is complaining of severe muscle cramping and joint pain. During your examination, you notice that his ECG shows a significant arrhythmia. What do you suspect?
   a. Influenza
   b. Recurrence of leukemia
   c. Low white blood cell count
   d. Tumor lysis syndrome

36. What is the most common cause of Cushing syndrome in an infant or toddler?
   a. Adrenal tumor
   b. Kidney disease
   c. Diabetes
   d. Pituitary tumor

37. A 10-year-old boy comes to the ER with a generalized red rash that feels like sandpaper. Upon examination, you note that his tongue appears swollen with a white coating through which the red papillae protrude. He is complaining of a sore throat, fever, headache, and abdominal pain with nausea and vomiting. What do you suspect?
   a. Rheumatic fever
   b. Fifth disease
   c. Scarlet fever
   d. Chickenpox

38. A 12-year-old boy arrives in the ER with acute onset of severe pain in the scrotal area, with no history of trauma. Upon examination, you note that the scrotum is swollen and has a bruised appearance, with one test is higher than the other and a transverse orientation. What do you suspect?

a. Acute hydrocele
b. Hemangioma
c. Testicular torsion
d. Pyocele

39. A 14-year-old girl comes to the ER with severe pain in her calf, and a history of falling several hours ago during tennis. The skin over the area appears pale, shiny, and swollen. She states that her leg is very weak. Any manipulation of the leg, foot, or toes results in excruciating pain. Pain medication and elevation of the limb provide no relief. What action do you take?

a. Apply ice and elevate extremity
b. Page the orthopedic surgeon
c. Page the physical therapist
d. Apply sequential stockings

40. A 15-year-old boy with a history of multiple bouts of tonsillitis and a recent tonsillectomy, with immediate postoperative bleed, arrives in the ER with nausea, vomiting, dizziness, and weakness. Which of the following would be the most appropriate first question?

a. What was the color and consistency of emesis?
b. Have you had any recent exposure to influenza?
c. What were your childhood illnesses?
d. Do you have a headache?

41. You have a 4-year-old boy admitted from a nearby resort with a near-drowning incident. He is coughing, complaining of chest pain with difficulty breathing, and seems unable to follow verbal commands. What do you suspect?

a. Posttraumatic stress
b. Dry drowning
c. Pneumonia
d. Bronchospasm

42. A young couple brings their 3-month-old son into the ER. They explain that he will not stop crying. During the physical examination, you note that the infant has excessive drooling and his limbs appear limp. Next, the infant vomits, appears lethargic, has difficulty breathing, and experiences a seizure. There is no rash and the temperature is normal. Which of the following do you suspect?

a. Meningitis
b. Teething
c. Strep throat
d. Shaken baby syndrome

43. A 7-year-old girl presents in the ER following a bicycle accident in which the handlebar punctured her abdomen. A CAT scan of the abdomen shows a possible laceration to the pancreas. Which of the following is accurate regarding this situation?

a. Surgical intervention or drain insertion will be required to remove hemorrhage and enzymatic spill
b. A pressure dressing to the wound plus antibiotic therapy will be all that is required
c. You should suction the wound with a sterile suction catheter to remove excess blood
d. A nasogastric tube is unnecessary in a child who may be going to surgery

44. A preprocedural assessment focuses on the respiratory and cardiovascular systems. AMPLE is an acronym used as a memory aid to gather the complete history of a patient preparing to undergo sedation. What does the "A" represent in this acronym?

a. Adverse reactions
b. Allergies
c. Anesthetic history
d. Age

45. What will you require for a patient during procedural sedation?

a. ECG, pulse oximeter
b. ECG, blood pressure monitor
c. Sequential stockings, pulse oximeter, ECG
d. ECG, pulse oximeter, blood pressure monitor

46. The nurse monitors the sedated patient during the procedure. At what point is the monitoring complete?

a. When the procedure ends
b. When the patient returns to preprocedure state
c. When the physician says to stop
d. 10 minutes postprocedure

47. You administer naloxone following a procedure in which the patient had sedation. One hour later the patient appears alert and oriented. Do you discharge the patient?

a. Yes, instruct the family that the patient should go home and sleep
b. Yes, instruct the family to monitor the patient and not allow them to sleep
c. No, keep the patient a minimum of 2 hours; he or she may relapse when the naloxone wears off
d. No, the patient may vomit and must stay to prevent nausea

48. You admit a 16-year-old girl who sustained severe trauma due to a motor vehicle accident in which her mother was the driver. The child has massive internal bleeding and must undergo exploratory surgery. Which is accurate regarding who signs the informed legal consent for the procedure?

a. The mother is clearly intoxicated but she can sign
b. The father is less intoxicated so he can sign
c. The patient is old enough to sign for herself
d. No consent is necessary since the situation is emergent

49. A young couple brings their 6-year-old boy into the ER with a high fever, nausea, and vomiting. The father states that they have no insurance. What law requires that hospital emergency departments provide emergency stabilization and appropriate medical screening exams for patients with emergency medical conditions and labor?

a. HIPAA
b. EMTALA
c. Health Care Reform Bill
d. EMS

50. Which of the following best describes "critical incident stress management debriefing"?

a. Structured group discussion to mitigate acute symptoms, assess need for follow-up, and provide sense of closure
b. One-on-one review of crisis situation, mitigate acute symptoms
c. Pre-crisis preparation, stress management education
d. Review of crisis response, assess technical performance, and adjust for future incidents

Answers and Explanations

1. D: The Pediatric Assessment Triangle (PAT) is the immediate observation prior to closely approaching the child. It includes Appearance to assess the mental status and muscle tone, Breathing through visual and audible clues, and Circulation by observing the skin color. Choice A is incorrect because the PAT should be initiated by observing the child from across the room; immediate close contact may cause fear and anxiety and skew the findings.

2. D: The purpose of the Pediatric Assessment Triangle is to determine the severity of the child's condition, if the child appears "sick" or "not sick," and to assess the need for immediate intervention. This is the initial evaluation and does not determine the diagnosis.

3. A: The child is assuming the sniffing position, which indicates that he is attempting to align the mouth, pharynx, and trachea to maintain an open airway. Cyanosis and increased respiratory rate are both signs of respiratory distress and possible impending respiratory failure. These findings denote that the child's condition is urgent and the nurse must proceed with rapid assessment of airway, breathing, and circulation. The child assumed the sniffing position as his response to his breathing difficulties, so having him lie down would make it more demanding on his respiratory system. Complete the history and physical after stabilizing him.

4. C: TICLS, pronounced tickles, refers to the assessment tool that evaluates the child's appearance.

5. B: The infant is head bobbing, which indicates difficulty with breathing. Sniffing refers to the position an older child assumes to align his mouth, pharynx, and trachea to increase airflow. Nasal flaring is a widening of the nares seen in infants with respiratory difficulties. Gasping is a short audible intake of air that indicates respiratory distress.

6. A: Elevation of the extremity is a first-aid measure to lessen the blood loss. Ascertaining the cause of the injury is not imperative at this stage. Checking the blood pressure and starting an IV are important steps, but do not lessen the rate of hemorrhage.

7. A: Epinephrine 0.5 mL of 1:1000 solution administered intramuscularly or subcutaneously is the correct dosage for anaphylaxis.

8. B: When reviewing the history of a patient using the mnemonic CIAMPEDS, the "C" refers to the "chief complaint." The possibility of contagion would be determined after establishing a diagnosis. Evaluate circulation and congenital abnormalities during the physical.

9. A: DCAP includes Deformities, Contusions, Abrasions, and Penetrations/Punctures. This mnemonic is useful during the physical examination of each section of the body. DCAP and BLS (Burns, Lacerations, Swelling or edema), plus TIC (Tenderness, Instability, and Crepitus) assess physical defects. Delusions, concussions, apprehension, and psychosis refer to mental conditions, not physical. Dyspnea, capillary refill, appearance, pallor, disability, circulation, airway, and pulse are observed or evaluated during a physical, but are not specifically named in this mnemonic.

10. B: Altered mental status, fever, drooling, and difficulty swallowing require medical attention within 10 minutes. These signs denote an emergent condition that could be life-threatening.

11. B: Bluish discoloration around the umbilicus, known as Cullen sign, may signify an intra-abdominal or retroperitoneal hemorrhage. Kehr sign refers to pain in the upper left quadrant radiating to the left shoulder as the result of blood or bile that is free in the abdomen, causing irritation of the diaphragm. Purpura is the term for reddish-purple, nonblanchable patches on the skin, which are larger than 0.5 cm in diameter. Petechiae are small reddish-purple spots on the skin, less than 0.5 cm in diameter. Both purpura and petechiae appear because of intravascular defects or infection.

12. A: Anyone who is accompanying the child may answer the questions regarding the patient's history, although the parent or guardian may be able to supply more details when they are available to interview.

13. C: When obtaining the history on an infant or toddler, it is important to determine birth information such as mother's age, length of gestation, weight at birth, congenital aberrations, and complications of pregnancy or delivery. Blood type, history of siblings, and known allergies may be part of any patient's assessment, but birth history is important information for infants and toddlers.

14. C: OPQRST is the acronym used to evaluate pain.

15. B: In addition to the names of prescribed medications, it is imperative to include OTC supplements, route of administration, dosage per day, frequency, and the indication. The brand, generic equivalent, expiration date, and pharmacy are all extraneous information.

16. D: When observing the interaction of family members, it is important to determine the primary caregiver, coping mechanisms, and family dynamics. Interviewing the caregiver to establish any cultural influences, observations, or concerns they may have is important in assessing the complete history of the child.

17. D: IOI infusion is absorbed more quickly than subcutaneous or rectal routes, and at the same rate as IV. Health care providers can learn this technique with proper training, often in little as 60 seconds. The IOI route is adequate for blood draws for laboratory testing.

18. A: Infant paddles for defibrillation are appropriate for patients up to 1 year of age or 10 kg. If infant paddles are not available, larger paddles may work, but use caution to prevent contact between the two.

19. B: The use of an improper gel, cream, paste, or pad may result in burns or sparks and could cause a fire, especially when defibrillating in an oxygen-rich area. Prior to applying paddles to the chest, the skin should be dry; damp skin may cause an uneven delivery of the current. An inadequate amount of conductive material may interfere with current delivery and result in burns to the skin. An excessive amount of conductive material could lead to arcing between the paddles and poor delivery of current to the heart muscle.

20. C: If peripheral sites are unavailable and large amounts of fluids will be required, use a central venous line. The frontal scalp vein and jugular vein may be accessible, but in an unstable patient, these sites are unreliable if CPR is necessary. The cephalic vein is peripheral and, in this situation, not available.

21. B: If the child is combative, efforts to immobilize her may result in spinal injury. Encourage the parents or guardians to hold her in a position that will prevent misalignment, and then apply a properly fitting cervical collar. Do not allow her freedom to move at will because of the risk of further damage. The weight of sand bags and IV bags are not appropriate for cervical injury, and could result in cervical misalignment.

22. B: Prior to initiating treatment on a child who has ingested a chemical, call the poison control center. Wear protective clothing. Do not take time to try to attain a specific neutralizing agent. Rinse any external chemicals with copious amounts of room temperature or cool water.

23. C: Bradycardia and pupillary changes are indicators of increased intracranial pressure (ICP). Increased pulse pressures with irregular pulse and respirations herald ICP. Clear nasal drainage may be the result of a leakage of cerebrospinal fluid due to a head injury, but is not a sign of ICP.

24. A: The first maneuver you perform is to position the infant over your arm, face down, supporting his head and neck. His head should be lower than his body. Next, deliver 5 back blows between the shoulder blades. If the object does not come out, proceed in positioning him on his back with his head lower than his body. Perform chest thrusts one finger width below the nipple line. Check his mouth and if the object is visible, remove it. Do not perform a blind finger sweep.

25. B: Mediastinal shift is the term used for the movement of the major blood vessels to the side opposite a pneumothorax chest injury. Tracheal deviation, or shifting of the trachea to the side opposite the injury, may accompany a mediastinal shift. Simple pneumothorax is the term used for a chest injury in which air enters the chest cavity through an opening in the chest wall. A tension pneumothorax is a critical situation in which the lung collapses completely, resulting in mediastinal shift and possible tracheal deviation, leading to shock.

26. C: When respiratory arrest is imminent, the pulse rate drops (bradycardia). The child may become drowsy or confused, there is an absence of wheezing, chest movements become paradoxical, and there is an absence of pulsus paradoxus.

27. B: The child should be kept as calm as possible, so IV insertion should not be attempted since the child is having mild symptoms. Application of pulse oximetry is necessary to evaluate the effectiveness of the respirations. Apply oxygen by a means that is least intrusive to the child. Allow the child to assume a position that is most comfortable for him.

28. B: The most important diagnostic tool for assessing a child with a suspected seizure is a complete history. A detailed description of the entire episode, including any pre-seizure symptoms or signs, type of motor activity or autonomic indicators (eg, drooling, incontinence), medical history, exposure to toxins, head trauma, illness or fever, hypoglycemia, breath holding, or diabetes, will help determine the type and possibly the focal point of the seizure. When performing the physical exam, it is important to note any oral injuries, head wounds or other trauma, incontinence, and any indication of poisoning, alcohol, burns, or the presence of a medical ID. A high fever may be the cause of the seizure, but the complete history is necessary before determining a diagnosis. Postictal confusion or somnolence may follow a seizure, and are components of the thorough history of the episode.

29. A: This infant's symptoms point to necrotizing enterocolitis, the death of intestinal tissue. This newborn's history of premature birth and having had blood transfusions increases the chances for

this condition. Intussusception most often occurs in infants between 5 months and 1 year of age and the symptoms include pulling of the legs up toward the stomach (colicky pain) accompanied by loud crying, "currant jelly" stool, and bilious vomiting. Intestinal obstruction presents with persistent vomiting, abdominal pain, and distention. Infant acid reflux symptoms include spitting up, irritability during feedings, coughing, wheezing, and crying after feedings when placed on back.

30. B: Brown- or reddish-tinged urine indicates hematuria, and foaming points to protein in the urine. The appearance of the urine plus swelling of the face, ankles, and feet indicates possible kidney disease. Dehydration could cause concentrated urine that may appear darker than normal, but not foamy. Heart disease may cause edema, but this combination of the dark, foamy urine with the edema would more likely denote a kidney problem. Symptoms of urethral obstruction include the inability to pass urine, or a urine stream that is very limited, and pain in the bladder area.

31. C: The main reason cat bites are difficult to treat is that they cause puncture wounds. The depth of the puncture wound leads to inefficient cleansing; the outcome is a high rate of infection. Tissue avulsion, bony penetration, and skull injury are more frequently the consequence of dog bites.

32. C: The ingestion of wild mushrooms can be life-threatening, and should never be done except by an expert in this type of botany. Several types of mushrooms can cause severe toxicity leading to liver and kidney failure and death. Since the first symptoms of mushroom poisoning are often diarrhea and vomiting, admit this child for further testing. Identification of the type of mushroom is important. Contact poison control.

33. D: Sickle cell anemia is a disease frequently seen in the African-American community, and is inherited as an autosomal recessive condition. Swelling of the fingers and/or toes and an enlarged spleen are common symptoms of this disease. Lymphoma, kidney disease, and mononucleosis may share some of the symptoms of edema and splenomegaly, but this combination of factors points to sickle cell anemia.

34. C: The presence of blood in the anterior chamber of the eye is hyphema. Conjunctivitis is the irritation of the covering of the sclera of the eye, the conjunctiva. Patients with retinal detachment often complain of a "curtain falling" over the field of vision. The retina is not externally visible. In order to diagnose a retinal detachment, the physician would need to dilate the pupils and examine the retinal of the eye with an indirect ophthalmoscope. A cataract is a condition in which the lens of the eye, which is located posterior to the iris and pupil, becomes opaque.

35. D: The boy has a history of chemotherapy that can cause tumor lysis syndrome. Hyperuricemia, hyperkalemia, and hypocalcemia can cause cardiac arrhythmias, muscle cramps, and joint pain. These conditions, along with hyperphosphatemia, can lead to kidney failure or a fatal arrhythmia in a post chemotherapy patient. Common symptoms of influenza are fever, chills, sore throat, and generalized body pains. Recurrence of leukemia would involve enlarged lymph nodes and possibly the spleen or liver, joint pain, fevers or night sweats, bleeding or bruising easily, weakness, and weight loss. A low white blood cell count (leukopenia) may be the result of chemotherapy, but would not cause all of these symptoms.

36. A: Cushing syndrome in an infant or toddler is most commonly the result of an adrenal tumor. It does not involve the pancreas (diabetes) or the kidneys. However, in children older than 7 years, the most common cause of Cushing syndrome is an ACTH-secreting pituitary adenoma.

37. C: This patient has the classic signs and symptoms of Scarlet fever, including the rash that feels like sandpaper, the strawberry tongue that has a white coating with the red papillae showing through, sore throat, and possible GI upset. Rheumatic fever follows a few weeks after an episode of strep throat, and involves multiple joint redness, swelling, and pain. Other symptoms may include fever, small painless nodules under the skin, chest pain, palpitations, slightly raised ragged rash, shortness of breath, and fatigue. Fifth disease signs are bright red patches on both cheeks, followed by a lacy rash on the arms and legs, which spreads to the trunk and buttocks within a couple of days. Chickenpox rash appears over the entire body and consists of papules, pustules, and vesicles. The child may have a fever, cough, itching, and abdominal pain.

38. C: Testicular torsion presents with a sudden onset of severe pain in the scrotal area with no history of trauma, erythema, and scrotal swelling. The extremely tender, high-riding testis with abnormal transverse orientation are classic symptoms. Scrotal enlargement is the main symptom of hydrocele with mild discomfort. Hemangioma of the scrotum is a rare condition that presents with a painless swelling in one testicle. A pyocele is similar to a hydrocele but contains purulent material, and is frequently subsequent to an injury.

39. B: A patient with the history of an injury to an extremity, followed by extreme pain, paleness, and weakness in that limb, may have compartment syndrome. This emergency may require immediate surgery, so the first action should be to page an orthopedic surgeon. Elevation of the limb may be appropriate, but ice may decrease the circulation. Physical therapy is not appropriate at this time. Sequential stockings would cause increased pain and possibly add to the injury.

40. A: The boy has a history of a recent tonsillectomy with multiple bouts of tonsillitis and postoperative hemorrhage. His current symptoms could be another hemorrhage. Swallowing blood from a postoperative tonsillectomy hemorrhage can cause nausea, vomiting, weakness, and dizziness from blood loss. The color and consistency of the emesis is important for determining the presence of blood. The other questions may follow, but it is imperative to ascertain if the boy is actively bleeding.

41. B: Dry drowning is an extremely serious condition, which may lead to death. In this situation, the lungs lose their ability to extract oxygen from inhaled air. It is frequently the result of a laryngospasm, an involuntary contraction of the laryngeal cords when exposed to even a small amount of liquid. This closing of the cords prevents oxygen from entering the lungs, but since the heart continues to beat, a small amount of blood may enter the airspace of the lungs. This can lead to hypoxia, and the victim may drown in his own fluids. Symptoms of dry drowning in a child include a persistent cough following the inhalation of any amount of liquid, chest pain, confusion, extreme fatigue, and vomiting. Posttraumatic stress symptoms consist of anxiety related to a traumatic experience, reliving of the episode, avoidance, and hypervigilance. Pneumonia and bronchitis may follow a dry drowning as complications, but the child's immediate history points to dry drowning.

42. D: This infant has symptoms of shaken baby syndrome. Meningitis symptoms in an infant this age may include lack of appetite, lethargy or irritability, a bulging fontanelle, and a high-pitched cry. Teething may cause drooling with swelling of the gums, but does not cause the series of symptoms and signs this infant is experiencing.

43. A: Laceration of the pancreas requires surgical intervention to evacuate intra-abdominal blood plus enzymatic contents, which are toxic to adjacent organs. The insertion of a drain to evacuate

any further leakage of pancreatic enzymes may be necessary. The physician most likely will order antibiotics to prevent infection; surgical intervention with drain insertion is necessary. The ER nurse should not insert a suction catheter blindly into the wound since this may cause further injury. A nasogastric tube is frequently necessary since an injured child often swallows large amounts of air, which can lead to gastric distention.

44. B: AMPLE stands for Allergies, Medications, Past medical history, Last oral intake, and Events leading to the procedure. Adverse reactions, anesthetic history, and age are important and fall under these broader headings.

45. D: A patient undergoing sedation for a procedure needs an ECG, blood pressure monitor, and pulse oximeter. The nurse monitors the heart rate, respirations, oxygen saturation, and blood pressure every 5 to 10 minutes, depending on the level of sedation.

46. B: Patients react differently to sedation. Monitor the patient until he or she returns to his or her preanesthetic state; since this varies with each person, there is no set time to end monitoring.

47. C: Sedatives have a longer effect than naloxone and may resedate the patient when the effects of the naloxone end. Monitor for at least 2 hours after the administration of naloxone. Do not discharge a patient who receives naloxone until the period in which resedation is possible has passed. The resedated patient may need assistance with breathing; monitor until the sedation period has passed.

48. D: When both parents are intoxicated, the patient is a minor, and the situation is a true emergency, surgery may proceed without an informed consent. According to MedLaw.com, a resource for health law, "Informed consent must be obtained and the informed consent form must be placed in the patient's medical record, prior to surgery, except in the case of emergency surgery."

49. B: EMTALA, the Emergency Medical Treatment and Labor Act of 1986, ensures that emergency departments assess and stabilize patients regardless of their ability to pay. The most well-known portion of the HIPAA regulation is the privacy section, which ensures that a patient's medical records remain private. The health care reform bill refers to changes made in the managed care medical insurance system. EMS is the abbreviation for emergency medical services.

50. A: A critical incident stress management debriefing refers to the process of a structured group discussion, held within 1 to 10 days of a crisis, designed to resolve acute symptoms, evaluate the need for follow-up, and bring closure to the incident. Debriefing indicates that the crisis is in the past, so pre-crisis preparation is not part of this session. One-on-one sessions may follow this initial debriefing, but are not part of it. Assessment of the response to the crisis is a separate issue; this process is to relieve the stress the incident has caused for the staff members.

Secret Key #1 - Time is Your Greatest Enemy

Pace Yourself

Wear a watch. At the beginning of the test, check the time (or start a chronometer on your watch to count the minutes), and check the time after every few questions to make sure you are "on schedule."

If you are forced to speed up, do it efficiently. Usually one or more answer choices can be eliminated without too much difficulty. Above all, don't panic. Don't speed up and just begin guessing at random choices. By pacing yourself, and continually monitoring your progress against your watch, you will always know exactly how far ahead or behind you are with your available time. If you find that you are one minute behind on the test, don't skip one question without spending any time on it, just to catch back up. Take 15 fewer seconds on the next four questions, and after four questions you'll have caught back up. Once you catch back up, you can continue working each problem at your normal pace.

Furthermore, don't dwell on the problems that you were rushed on. If a problem was taking up too much time and you made a hurried guess, it must be difficult. The difficult questions are the ones you are most likely to miss anyway, so it isn't a big loss. It is better to end with more time than you need than to run out of time.

Lastly, sometimes it is beneficial to slow down if you are constantly getting ahead of time. You are always more likely to catch a careless mistake by working more slowly than quickly, and among very high-scoring test takers (those who are likely to have lots of time left over), careless errors affect the score more than mastery of material.

Secret Key #2 - Guessing is not Guesswork

You probably know that guessing is a good idea. Unlike other standardized tests, there is no penalty for getting a wrong answer. Even if you have no idea about a question, you still have a 20-25% chance of getting it right.

Most test takers do not understand the impact that proper guessing can have on their score. Unless you score extremely high, guessing will significantly contribute to your final score.

Monkeys Take the Test

What most test takers don't realize is that to insure that 20-25% chance, you have to guess randomly. If you put 20 monkeys in a room to take this test, assuming they answered once per question and behaved themselves, on average they would get 20-25% of the questions correct. Put 20 test takers in the room, and the average will be much lower among guessed questions. Why?

1. The test writers intentionally write deceptive answer choices that "look" right. A test taker has no idea about a question, so he picks the "best looking" answer, which is often wrong. The monkey has no idea what looks good and what doesn't, so it will consistently be right

about 20-25% of the time.

2. Test takers will eliminate answer choices from the guessing pool based on a hunch or intuition. Simple but correct answers often get excluded, leaving a 0% chance of being correct. The monkey has no clue, and often gets lucky with the best choice.

This is why the process of elimination endorsed by most test courses is flawed and detrimental to your performance. Test takers don't guess; they make an ignorant stab in the dark that is usually worse than random.

$5 Challenge

Let me introduce one of the most valuable ideas of this course—the $5 challenge:

You only mark your "best guess" if you are willing to bet $5 on it.
You only eliminate choices from guessing if you are willing to bet $5 on it.

Why $5? Five dollars is an amount of money that is small yet not insignificant, and can really add up fast (20 questions could cost you $100). Likewise, each answer choice on one question of the test will have a small impact on your overall score, but it can really add up to a lot of points in the end.

The process of elimination IS valuable. The following shows your chance of guessing it right:

If you eliminate wrong answer choices until only this many remain:	Chance of getting it correct:
1	100%
2	50%
3	33%

However, if you accidentally eliminate the right answer or go on a hunch for an incorrect answer, your chances drop dramatically—to 0%. By guessing among all the answer choices, you are GUARANTEED to have a shot at the right answer.

That's why the $5 test is so valuable. If you give up the advantage and safety of a pure guess, it had better be worth the risk.

What we still haven't covered is how to be sure that whatever guess you make is truly random. Here's the easiest way:

Always pick the first answer choice among those remaining.

Such a technique means that you have decided, **before you see a single test question**, exactly how you are going to guess, and since the order of choices tells you nothing about which one is correct, this guessing technique is perfectly random.

This section is not meant to scare you away from making educated guesses or eliminating choices; you just need to define when a choice is worth eliminating. The $5 test, along with a pre-defined random guessing strategy, is the best way to make sure you reap all of the benefits of guessing.

Secret Key #3 - Practice Smarter, Not Harder

Many test takers delay the test preparation process because they dread the awful amounts of practice time they think necessary to succeed on the test. We have refined an effective method that will take you only a fraction of the time.

There are a number of "obstacles" in the path to success. Among these are answering questions, finishing in time, and mastering test-taking strategies. All must be executed on the day of the test at peak performance, or your score will suffer. The test is a mental marathon that has a large impact on your future.

Just like a marathon runner, it is important to work your way up to the full challenge. So first you just worry about questions, and then time, and finally strategy:

Success Strategy

1. Find a good source for practice tests.
2. If you are willing to make a larger time investment, consider using more than one study guide. Often the different approaches of multiple authors will help you "get" difficult concepts.
3. Take a practice test with no time constraints, with all study helps, "open book." Take your time with questions and focus on applying strategies.
4. Take a practice test with time constraints, with all guides, "open book."
5. Take a final practice test without open material and with time limits.

If you have time to take more practice tests, just repeat step 5. By gradually exposing yourself to the full rigors of the test environment, you will condition your mind to the stress of test day and maximize your success.

Secret Key #4 - Prepare, Don't Procrastinate

Let me state an obvious fact: if you take the test three times, you will probably get three different scores. This is due to the way you feel on test day, the level of preparedness you have, and the version of the test you see. Despite the test writers' claims to the contrary, some versions of the test WILL be easier for you than others.

Since your future depends so much on your score, you should maximize your chances of success. In order to maximize the likelihood of success, you've got to prepare in advance. This means taking practice tests and spending time learning the information and test taking strategies you will need to succeed.

Never go take the actual test as a "practice" test, expecting that you can just take it again if you need to. Take all the practice tests you can on your own, but when you go to take the official test, be prepared, be focused, and do your best the first time!

Secret Key #5 - Test Yourself

Everyone knows that time is money. There is no need to spend too much of your time or too little of your time preparing for the test. You should only spend as much of your precious time preparing as is necessary for you to get the score you need.

Once you have taken a practice test under real conditions of time constraints, then you will know if you are ready for the test or not.

If you have scored extremely high the first time that you take the practice test, then there is not much point in spending countless hours studying. You are already there.

Benchmark your abilities by retaking practice tests and seeing how much you have improved. Once you consistently score high enough to guarantee success, then you are ready.

If you have scored well below where you need, then knuckle down and begin studying in earnest. Check your improvement regularly through the use of practice tests under real conditions. Above all, don't worry, panic, or give up. The key is perseverance!

Then, when you go to take the test, remain confident and remember how well you did on the practice tests. If you can score high enough on a practice test, then you can do the same on the real thing.

General Strategies

The most important thing you can do is to ignore your fears and jump into the test immediately. Do not be overwhelmed by any strange-sounding terms. You have to jump into the test like jumping into a pool—all at once is the easiest way.

Make Predictions

As you read and understand the question, try to guess what the answer will be. Remember that several of the answer choices are wrong, and once you begin reading them, your mind will immediately become cluttered with answer choices designed to throw you off. Your mind is typically the most focused immediately after you have read the question and digested its contents. If you can, try to predict what the correct answer will be. You may be surprised at what you can predict.

Quickly scan the choices and see if your prediction is in the listed answer choices. If it is, then you can be quite confident that you have the right answer. It still won't hurt to check the other answer choices, but most of the time, you've got it!

Answer the Question

It may seem obvious to only pick answer choices that answer the question, but the test writers can create some excellent answer choices that are wrong. Don't pick an answer just because it sounds right, or you believe it to be true. It MUST answer the question. Once you've made your selection, always go back and check it against the question and make sure that you didn't misread the question and that the answer choice does answer the question posed.

Benchmark
After you read the first answer choice, decide if you think it sounds correct or not. If it doesn't, move on to the next answer choice. If it does, mentally mark that answer choice. This doesn't mean that you've definitely selected it as your answer choice, it just means that it's the best you've seen thus far. Go ahead and read the next choice. If the next choice is worse than the one you've already selected, keep going to the next answer choice. If the next choice is better than the choice you've already selected, mentally mark the new answer choice as your best guess.

The first answer choice that you select becomes your standard. Every other answer choice must be benchmarked against that standard. That choice is correct until proven otherwise by another answer choice beating it out. Once you've decided that no other answer choice seems as good, do one final check to ensure that your answer choice answers the question posed.

Valid Information
Don't discount any of the information provided in the question. Every piece of information may be necessary to determine the correct answer. None of the information in the question is there to throw you off (while the answer choices will certainly have information to throw you off). If two seemingly unrelated topics are discussed, don't ignore either. You can be confident there is a relationship, or it wouldn't be included in the question, and you are probably going to have to determine what is that relationship to find the answer.

Avoid "Fact Traps"
Don't get distracted by a choice that is factually true. Your search is for the answer that answers the question. Stay focused and don't fall for an answer that is true but irrelevant. Always go back to the question and make sure you're choosing an answer that actually answers the question and is not just a true statement. An answer can be factually correct, but it MUST answer the question asked. Additionally, two answers can both be seemingly correct, so be sure to read all of the answer choices, and make sure that you get the one that BEST answers the question.

Milk the Question
Some of the questions may throw you completely off. They might deal with a subject you have not been exposed to, or one that you haven't reviewed in years. While your lack of knowledge about the subject will be a hindrance, the question itself can give you many clues that will help you find the correct answer. Read the question carefully and look for clues. Watch particularly for adjectives and nouns describing difficult terms or words that you don't recognize. Regardless of whether you completely understand a word or not, replacing it with a synonym, either provided or one you more familiar with, may help you to understand what the questions are asking. Rather than wracking your mind about specific detailed information concerning a difficult term or word, try to use mental substitutes that are easier to understand.

The Trap of Familiarity
Don't just choose a word because you recognize it. On difficult questions, you may not recognize a number of words in the answer choices. The test writers don't put "make-believe" words on the test, so don't think that just because you only recognize all the words in one answer choice that that answer choice must be correct. If you only recognize words in one answer choice, then focus on that one. Is it correct? Try your best to determine if it is correct. If it is, that's great. If not, eliminate it. Each word and answer choice you eliminate increases your chances of getting the question correct, even if you then have to guess among the unfamiliar choices.

Eliminate Answers
Eliminate choices as soon as you realize they are wrong. But be careful! Make sure you consider all

of the possible answer choices. Just because one appears right, doesn't mean that the next one won't be even better! The test writers will usually put more than one good answer choice for every question, so read all of them. Don't worry if you are stuck between two that seem right. By getting down to just two remaining possible choices, your odds are now 50/50. Rather than wasting too much time, play the odds. You are guessing, but guessing wisely because you've been able to knock out some of the answer choices that you know are wrong. If you are eliminating choices and realize that the last answer choice you are left with is also obviously wrong, don't panic. Start over and consider each choice again. There may easily be something that you missed the first time and will realize on the second pass.

Tough Questions

If you are stumped on a problem or it appears too hard or too difficult, don't waste time. Move on! Remember though, if you can quickly check for obviously incorrect answer choices, your chances of guessing correctly are greatly improved. Before you completely give up, at least try to knock out a couple of possible answers. Eliminate what you can and then guess at the remaining answer choices before moving on.

Brainstorm

If you get stuck on a difficult question, spend a few seconds quickly brainstorming. Run through the complete list of possible answer choices. Look at each choice and ask yourself, "Could this answer the question satisfactorily?" Go through each answer choice and consider it independently of the others. By systematically going through all possibilities, you may find something that you would otherwise overlook. Remember though that when you get stuck, it's important to try to keep moving.

Read Carefully

Understand the problem. Read the question and answer choices carefully. Don't miss the question because you misread the terms. You have plenty of time to read each question thoroughly and make sure you understand what is being asked. Yet a happy medium must be attained, so don't waste too much time. You must read carefully, but efficiently.

Face Value

When in doubt, use common sense. Always accept the situation in the problem at face value. Don't read too much into it. These problems will not require you to make huge leaps of logic. The test writers aren't trying to throw you off with a cheap trick. If you have to go beyond creativity and make a leap of logic in order to have an answer choice answer the question, then you should look at the other answer choices. Don't overcomplicate the problem by creating theoretical relationships or explanations that will warp time or space. These are normal problems rooted in reality. It's just that the applicable relationship or explanation may not be readily apparent and you have to figure things out. Use your common sense to interpret anything that isn't clear.

Prefixes

If you're having trouble with a word in the question or answer choices, try dissecting it. Take advantage of every clue that the word might include. Prefixes and suffixes can be a huge help. Usually they allow you to determine a basic meaning. Pre- means before, post- means after, pro - is positive, de- is negative. From these prefixes and suffixes, you can get an idea of the general meaning of the word and try to put it into context. Beware though of any traps. Just because con- is the opposite of pro-, doesn't necessarily mean congress is the opposite of progress!

Hedge Phrases

Watch out for critical hedge phrases, led off with words such as "likely," "may," "can," "sometimes," "often," "almost," "mostly," "usually," "generally," "rarely," and "sometimes." Question writers insert these hedge phrases to cover every possibility. Often an answer choice will be wrong simply because it leaves no room for exception. Unless the situation calls for them, avoid answer choices that have definitive words like "exactly," and "always."

Switchback Words
Stay alert for "switchbacks." These are the words and phrases frequently used to alert you to shifts in thought. The most common switchback word is "but." Others include "although," "however," "nevertheless," "on the other hand," "even though," "while," "in spite of," "despite," and "regardless of."

New Information
Correct answer choices will rarely have completely new information included. Answer choices typically are straightforward reflections of the material asked about and will directly relate to the question. If a new piece of information is included in an answer choice that doesn't even seem to relate to the topic being asked about, then that answer choice is likely incorrect. All of the information needed to answer the question is usually provided for you in the question. You should not have to make guesses that are unsupported or choose answer choices that require unknown information that cannot be reasoned from what is given.

Time Management
On technical questions, don't get lost on the technical terms. Don't spend too much time on any one question. If you don't know what a term means, then odds are you aren't going to get much further since you don't have a dictionary. You should be able to immediately recognize whether or not you know a term. If you don't, work with the other clues that you have—the other answer choices and terms provided—but don't waste too much time trying to figure out a difficult term that you don't know.

Contextual Clues
Look for contextual clues. An answer can be right but not the correct answer. The contextual clues will help you find the answer that is most right and is correct. Understand the context in which a phrase or statement is made. This will help you make important distinctions.

Don't Panic
Panicking will not answer any questions for you; therefore, it isn't helpful. When you first see the question, if your mind goes blank, take a deep breath. Force yourself to mechanically go through the steps of solving the problem using the strategies you've learned.

Pace Yourself
Don't get clock fever. It's easy to be overwhelmed when you're looking at a page full of questions, your mind is full of random thoughts and feeling confused, and the clock is ticking down faster than you would like. Calm down and maintain the pace that you have set for yourself. As long as you are on track by monitoring your pace, you are guaranteed to have enough time for yourself. When you get to the last few minutes of the test, it may seem like you won't have enough time left, but if you only have as many questions as you should have left at that point, then you're right on track!

Answer Selection
The best way to pick an answer choice is to eliminate all of those that are wrong, until only one is left and confirm that is the correct answer. Sometimes though, an answer choice may immediately look right. Be careful! Take a second to make sure that the other choices are not equally obvious. Don't make a hasty mistake. There are only two times that you should stop before checking other answers. First is when you are positive that the answer choice you have selected is correct. Second

is when time is almost out and you have to make a quick guess!

Check Your Work

Since you will probably not know every term listed and the answer to every question, it is important that you get credit for the ones that you do know. Don't miss any questions through careless mistakes. If at all possible, try to take a second to look back over your answer selection and make sure you've selected the correct answer choice and haven't made a costly careless mistake (such as marking an answer choice that you didn't mean to mark). The time it takes for this quick double check should more than pay for itself in caught mistakes.

Beware of Directly Quoted Answers

Sometimes an answer choice will repeat word for word a portion of the question or reference section. However, beware of such exact duplication. It may be a trap! More than likely, the correct choice will paraphrase or summarize a point, rather than being exactly the same wording.

Slang

Scientific sounding answers are better than slang ones. An answer choice that begins "To compare the outcomes…" is much more likely to be correct than one that begins "Because some people insisted…"

Extreme Statements

Avoid wild answers that throw out highly controversial ideas that are proclaimed as established fact. An answer choice that states the "process should be used in certain situations, if…" is much more likely to be correct than one that states the "process should be discontinued completely." The first is a calm rational statement and doesn't even make a definitive, uncompromising stance, using a hedge word "if" to provide wiggle room, whereas the second choice is a radical idea and far more extreme.

Answer Choice Families

When you have two or more answer choices that are direct opposites or parallels, one of them is usually the correct answer. For instance, if one answer choice states "x increases" and another answer choice states "x decreases" or "y increases," then those two or three answer choices are very similar in construction and fall into the same family of answer choices. A family of answer choices consists of two or three answer choices, very similar in construction, but often with directly opposite meanings. Usually the correct answer choice will be in that family of answer choices. The "odd man out" or answer choice that doesn't seem to fit the parallel construction of the other answer choices is more likely to be incorrect.

Special Report: Additional Bonus Material

Due to our efforts to try to keep this book to a manageable length, we've created a link that will give you access to all of your additional bonus material.

Please visit http://www.mometrix.com/bonus948/cpen to access the information.